Diagnosis of
fetal abnormalities
The 18–23-week scan

Diploma in Fetal Medicine Series
Series Editor: K. H. Nicolaides

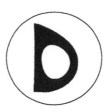

Diagnosis of fetal abnormalities
The 18–23-week scan

Gianluigi Pilu & Kypros H. Nicolaides

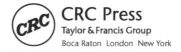

CRC Press
Taylor & Francis Group
Boca Raton London New York

CRC Press is an imprint of the
Taylor & Francis Group, an **informa** business

CRC Press
Taylor & Francis Group
6000 Broken Sound Parkway NW, Suite 300
Boca Raton, FL 33487-2742

First issued in paperback 2019

© 1999 by Taylor & Francis Group, LLC
CRC Press is an imprint of Taylor & Francis Group, an Informa business
Typeset by AMA DataSet Ltd, Preston, UK

No claim to original U.S. Government works

ISBN-13: 978-1-85070-492-8 (hbk)
ISBN-13: 978-0-367-39968-9 (pbk)

A CIP record for this book is available from the British Library.

**Visit the Taylor & Francis Web site at
http://www.taylorandfrancis.com**

**and the CRC Press Web site at
http://www.crcpress.com**

Contents

Introduction

Ultrasound is the main diagnostic tool in the prenatal detection of congenital abnormalities. It allows examination of the external and internal anatomy of the fetus and the detection of not only major defects but also of subtle markers of chromosomal abnormalities and genetic syndromes. Although some women are at high risk of fetal abnormalities, either because of a family history or due to exposure to teratogens such as infection and various drugs, the vast majority of fetal abnormalities occur in the low-risk group. Consequently, ultrasound examination should be offered routinely to all pregnant women. The scan, which is usually performed at 18–23 weeks of pregnancy, should be carried out to a high standard and should include systematic examination of the fetus for the detection of both major and minor defects.

The Fetal Medicine Foundation, under the auspices of the International Society of Ultrasound in Obstetrics and Gynecology and the World Association of Perinatal Medicine, has introduced a process of training and certification to help establish high standards of scanning on an international basis. The Certificate of Competence in the 18–23-week scan is awarded to those sonographers that can perform the scan to a high standard and can demonstrate a good knowledge of a wide spectrum of fetal abnormalities.

This book, which summarizes the prevalence, etiology, prenatal sonographic features and prognosis for both common and rare fetal abnormalities, provides the basis of learning for the theoretical component of the Certificate of Competence in the 18–23-week scan.

1

Standard views for examination of the fetus

At the 18–23-week scan, the necessary views should be obtained to examine routinely the following organs:

(1) Skull   Examination of integrity and normal shape, and measurement of biparietal diameter and head circumference

(2) Brain   Examination of cerebral ventricles, choroid plexuses, mid-brain, posterior fossa (cerebellum and cisterna magna), and measurement of the anterior and posterior horns of the lateral ventricles

(3) Face   Examination of the profile, orbits and upper lip

(4) Neck   Measurement of nuchal fold thickness

(5) Spine   Examination both longitudinally and transversely

(6) Heart   Examination of rate and rhythm, four-chamber view, and outflow tracts

(7) Thorax   Examination of the shape of the thorax, the lungs and diaphragm

(8) Abdomen   Examination of the stomach, liver, kidneys, bladder, abdominal wall and umbilicus, and measurement of abdominal circumference

(9) Limbs   Examination of the femur, tibia and fibula, humerus, radius and ulna, hands and feet (including shape and echogenicity of long bones and movement of joints), and measurement of femur length

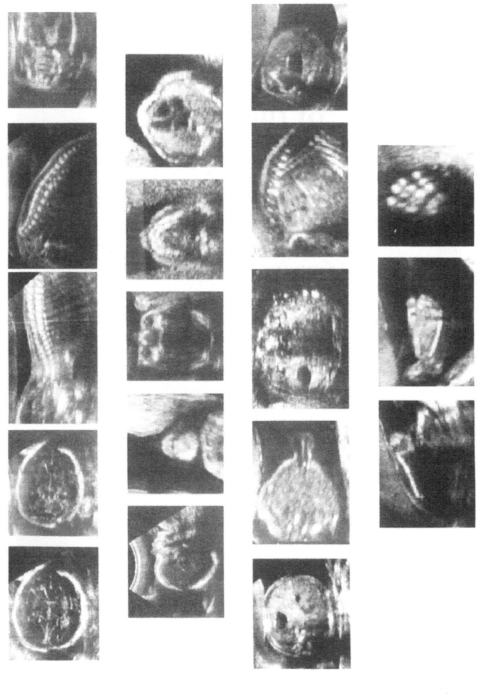

Figure 1 Standard views for examination of the fetus

4

2

Central nervous system

NORMAL SONOGRAPHIC ANATOMY

The fetal brain undergoes major developmental changes throughout pregnancy. At 7 weeks of gestation, a sonolucent area is seen in the cephalic pole, presumably representing the fluid-filled rhombencephalic vesicle. At 9 weeks, demonstration of the convoluted pattern of the three primary cerebral vesicles is feasible. From 11 weeks, the brightly echogenic choroid plexuses filling the large lateral ventricles are the most prominent intracranial structures. In the early second trimester, the lateral ventricles and choroid plexuses decrease in size relative to the brain mass.

Examination of the fetal brain can essentially be carried out by two transverse planes (see Figure 2, p. 15). A transverse scan at the level of the cavum septum pellucidum will demonstrate the lateral borders of the anterior horns, the medial and lateral borders of the posterior horns of the lateral ventricles, the choroid plexuses, the third ventricle and the Sylvian fissures; this view is used for measurement of the biparietal diameter (BPD), head circumference (HC), and width of the ventricles. The suboccipitobregmatic view allows examination of the mid-brain and posterior fossa; this view is used for measurement of the transverse cerebellar diameter (TCD) and cisterna magna.

Additional scanning planes along different orientations may be required from time to time to better define subtle details of intracranial anatomy in selected cases. Reverberation artifacts usually obscure the cerebral hemisphere close to the transducer. Visualization of both cerebral hemispheres would require sagittal and coronal planes that are often difficult to obtain and may require vaginal sonography. Luckily, unilateral cerebral lesions are rare and are often associated with a shift in the mid-line echo. Therefore, we adhere to the approach that, in standard examination, only one hemisphere is seen, and symmetry is assumed unless otherwise proven.

A sagittal and/or coronal view of the entire fetal spine should be obtained in each case (see Figure 4, p. 16). In the sagittal plane, the normal spine has a 'double railway' appearance and it is possible to appreciate the intact soft tissues above it. In the coronal plane, the three ossification centers of the vertebrae form three regular lines that tether down into the sacrum. These views are used to assess the integrity of the vertebrae (to rule out spina bifida) and the presence and regularity of the whole spine (to rule out sacral agenesis and scoliosis). Whether a systematic examination of each neural arch, from the cervical to the sacral region in the transverse plane, is necessary is debatable. This is certainly required for patients at high risk of neural tube defects. In low-risk patients, intact cerebral anatomy rules out more than 90% of cases of spina bifida and we believe that the longitudinal/coronal scan may suffice.

NEURAL TUBE DEFECTS

These include anencephaly, spina bifida and encephalocele. In anencephaly, there is absence of the cranial vault (acrania) with secondary degeneration of the brain. Encephaloceles are cranial defects, usually occipital, with herniated fluid-filled or brain-filled cysts. In spina bifida, the neural arch, usually in the lumbosacral region, is incomplete with secondary damage to the exposed nerves.

Prevalence

This is subject to large geographical and temporal variations; in the UK the prevalence is about 5 per 1000 births. Anencephaly and spina bifida, with an approximately equal prevalence, account for 95% of the cases and encephalocele for the remaining 5%.

Etiology

Chromosomal abnormalities, single mutant genes, and maternal diabetes mellitus or ingestion of teratogens, such as antiepileptic drugs, are implicated in about 10% of the cases. However, the precise etiology for the majority of these defects is unknown. When a parent or previous sibling has had a neural tube defect, the risk of recurrence is 5–10%. Periconceptual supplementation of the maternal diet with folate reduces by about half the risk of developing these defects.

Diagnosis

The diagnosis of anencephaly during the second trimester of pregnancy is based on the demonstration of absent cranial vault and cerebral hemispheres (see Figure 3, p. 15). However, the facial bones, brain stem and portions of the occipital bones and mid-brain are usually present. Associated spinal lesions are found in up to 50% of cases. In the first trimester, the diagnosis can be made after 11 weeks, when ossification of the skull normally occurs. Ultrasound reports have demonstrated that there is progression from acrania to exencephaly and finally anencephaly. In the first trimester, the pathognomonic feature is acrania, the brain being either entirely normal or at varying degrees of distortion and disruption.

Diagnosis of spina bifida requires the systematic examination of each neural arch, from the cervical to the sacral region, both transversely and longitudinally (see Figure 4, p. 16). In the transverse scan, the normal neural arch appears as a closed circle with an intact skin covering, whereas in spina bifida the arch is 'U'-shaped and there is an associated bulging meningocele (thin-walled cyst) or myelomeningocele. The extent of the defect and any associated kyphoscoliosis are best assessed in the longitudinal scan.

The diagnosis of spina bifida has been greatly enhanced by the recognition of associated abnormalities in the skull and brain. These abnormalities include frontal bone scalloping (lemon sign), and obliteration of the cisterna magna with either an 'absent' cerebellum or abnormal anterior curvature of the cerebellar hemispheres (banana sign). These easily recognizable alterations in skull and brain morphology are often more readily attainable than detailed spinal views. A variable degree of ventricular enlargement is present in virtually all cases of open spina bifida at birth, but in only about 70% of cases in the mid-trimester.

Encephaloceles are recognized as cranial defects with herniated fluid-filled or brain-filled cysts. They are most commonly found in an occipital location (75% of the cases), but alternative sites include the frontoethmoidal and parietal regions.

Prognosis

Anencephaly is fatal at or within hours of birth. In encephalocele, the prognosis is inversely related to the amount of herniated cerebral tissue. Overall, the neonatal mortality is about 40% and more that 80% of survivors are intellectually and neurologically handicapped. In spina bifida, the surviving infants are often severely handicapped, with paralysis in the lower limbs and double incontinence; despite the associated hydrocephalus requiring surgery, intelligence may be normal.

Fetal therapy

There is some experimental evidence that *in utero* closure of spina bifida may reduce the risk of handicap because the amniotic fluid in the third trimester is thought to be neurotoxic.

HYDROCEPHALUS AND VENTRICULOMEGALY

In hydrocephalus, there is a pathological increase in the size of the cerebral ventricles.

Prevalence

Hydrocephalus is found in about 2 per 1000 births. Ventriculomegaly (lateral ventricle diameter of 10 mm or more) is found in 1% of pregnancies at the 18–23-week scan. Therefore, the majority of fetuses with ventriculomegaly do not develop hydrocephalus.

Etiology

This may result from chromosomal and genetic abnormalities, intrauterine hemorrhage or congenital infection, although many cases have as yet no clear-cut etiology.

Diagnosis

Fetal hydrocephalus is diagnosed sonographically by the demonstration of abnormally dilated lateral cerebral ventricles (see Figure 5, p. 16). Certainly, before 24 weeks and particularly in cases of associated spina bifida, the head circumference may be small rather than large for gestation. A transverse scan of the fetal head at the level of the cavum septum pellucidum will demonstrate the dilated lateral ventricles, defined by a diameter of 10 mm or more. The choroid plexuses, which normally fill the lateral ventricles, are surrounded by fluid.

Prognosis

Fetal or perinatal death and neurodevelopment in survivors are strongly related to the presence of other malformations and chromosomal defects. Although mild ventriculomegaly (atrial width of 10–15 mm) is generally associated with a good prognosis, affected fetuses form the group with the highest incidence of chromosomal abnormalities (often trisomy 21). In addition, in a few cases with apparently isolated mild ventriculomegaly, there may be an underlying cerebral maldevelopment (such as lissencephaly) or destructive lesion (such as periventricular leukomalacia). Recent evidence suggests that, in about 10% of cases, there is mild to moderate neurodevelopmental delay.

Fetal therapy

There is some experimental evidence that *in utero* cerebrospinal fluid diversion may be beneficial. However, attempts in the 1980s to treat hydrocephalic fetuses by ventriculo–amniotic shunting have now been abandoned because of poor results, mainly because of inappropriate selection of patients. It is possible that intrauterine drainage may be beneficial if all intra- and extra-cerebral malformations and chromosomal defects are excluded, and if serial ultrasound scans demonstrate progressive ventriculomegaly.

HOLOPROSENCEPHALY

This is a spectrum of cerebral abnormalities resulting from incomplete cleavage of the forebrain. There are three types according to the degree of forebrain cleavage. The alobar type, which is the most severe, is characterized by a monoventricular cavity and fusion of the thalami. In the semilobar type, there is partial segmentation of the ventricles and cerebral hemispheres posteriorly with incomplete fusion of the thalami. In lobar holoprosencephaly, there is normal separation of the ventricles and thalami but absence of the septum pellucidum. The first two types are often accompanied by microcephaly and facial abnormalities.

Prevalence

Holoprosencephaly is found in about 1 per 10 000 births.

Etiology

Although in many cases the cause is a chromosomal abnormality (usually trisomy 13) or a genetic disorder with an autosomal dominant or recessive mode of transmission, in many cases the etiology is unknown. For sporadic, non-chromosomal holoprosencephaly, the empirical recurrence risk is 6%.

Diagnosis

In the standard transverse view of the fetal head for measurement of the biparietal diameter, there is a single dilated mid-line ventricle replacing the two lateral ventricles or partial segmentation of the ventricles (see Figure 6, p. 17). The alobar and semilobar types are often associated with facial defects, such as hypotelorism or cyclopia, facial cleft and nasal hypoplasia or proboscis.

Prognosis

Alobar and semilobar holoprosencephaly are lethal. Lobar holoprosencephaly is associated with mental retardation.

AGENESIS OF THE CORPUS CALLOSUM

The corpus callosum is a bundle of fibers that connects the two cerebral hemispheres. It develops at 12–18 weeks of gestation. Agenesis of the corpus callosum may be either complete or partial (usually affecting the posterior part).

Prevalence

Agenesis of the corpus callosum is found in about 5 per 1000 births.

Etiology

Agenesis of the corpus callosum may be due to maldevelopment or secondary to a destructive lesion. It is commonly associated with chromosomal abnormalities (usually trisomies 18, 13 and 8) and more than 100 genetic syndromes.

Diagnosis

The corpus callosum is not visible in the standard transverse views of the brain, but agenesis of the corpus callosum may be suspected by the absence of the cavum septum pellucidum and the 'teardrop' configuration of the lateral ventricles (enlargement of the posterior horns). Agenesis of the corpus callosum is demonstrated in the mid-coronal and mid-sagittal views, which may require vaginal sonography.

Prognosis

This depends on the underlying cause. In about 90% of those with apparently isolated agenesis of the corpus callosum, development is normal.

DANDY–WALKER COMPLEX

The Dandy–Walker complex refers to a spectrum of abnormalities of the cerebellar vermis, cystic dilatation of the fourth ventricle and enlargement of the cisterna magna. The condition is classified into:

(1) Dandy–Walker malformation (complete or partial agenesis of the cerebellar vermis and enlarged posterior fossa);

(2) Dandy–Walker variant (partial agenesis of the cerebellar vermis without enlargement of the posterior fossa); and

(3) Mega-cisterna magna (normal vermis and fourth ventricle).

Prevalence

Dandy–Walker malformation is found in about 1 per 30 000 births.

Etiology

The Dandy–Walker complex is a non-specific end-point of chromosomal abnormalities (usually trisomies 18 or 13 and triploidy), more than 50 genetic syndromes, congenital infection or teratogens such as warfarin, but it can also be an isolated finding.

Diagnosis

Ultrasonographically, the contents of the posterior fossa are visualized through a transverse suboccipitobregmatic section of the fetal head (see Figure 7, p. 18). In the Dandy–Walker malformation, there is cystic dilatation of the fourth ventricle with partial or complete agenesis of the vermis; in more than 50% of the cases there is associated hydrocephalus and other extracranial defects. Enlarged cisterna magna is diagnosed if the vertical distance from the vermis to the inner border of the skull is more than 10 mm. Prenatal diagnosis of isolated partial agenesis of the vermis is difficult and a false diagnosis can be made if the angle of insonation is too steep.

Prognosis

Dandy–Walker malformation is associated with a high postnatal mortality (about 20%) and a high incidence (more than 50%) of impaired intellectual and neurological development. Experience with apparently isolated partial agenesis of the vermis or enlarged cisterna magna is limited and the prognosis for these conditions is uncertain.

MICROCEPHALY

Microcephaly means small head and brain.

Prevalence

Microcephaly is found in about 1 per 1000 births.

Etiology

This may result from chromosomal and genetic abnormalities, fetal hypoxia, congenital infection, and exposure to radiation or other teratogens, such as maternal anticoagulation with warfarin. It is commonly found in the presence of other brain abnormalities, such as encephalocele or holoprosencephaly.

Diagnosis

The diagnosis is made by the demonstration of brain abnormalities, such as holoprosencephaly. In cases with apparently isolated microcephaly, it is necessary to demonstrate progressive decrease in the head-to-abdomen circumference ratio to below the 1st centile with advancing gestation. Such a diagnosis may not be apparent before the third trimester. In microcephaly, there is a typical disproportion between the size of the skull and the face. The brain is small, with the cerebral hemispheres affected to a greater extent than the mid-brain and posterior fossa.

Prognosis

This depends on the underlying cause, but in more than 50% of cases there is severe mental retardation.

MEGALENCEPHALY

Megalencephaly means large head and brain.

Prevalence

Megalencephaly is a very rare abnormality.

Etiology

This is usually familial with no adverse consequence. However, it may also be the consequence of genetic syndromes, such as Beckwith–Wiedemann syndrome, achondroplasia, neurofibromatosis, and tuberous sclerosis. Unilateral megalencephaly is a sporadic condition.

Diagnosis

The diagnosis is made by the demonstration of a head-to-abdomen circumference ratio above the 99th centile without evidence of hydrocephalus or intracranial masses. Unilateral megalencephaly is characterized by macrocrania, a shift in the mid-line echo, borderline enlargement of the lateral ventricle and atypical gyri of the affected hemisphere.

Prognosis

Isolated megalencephaly is usually an asymptomatic condition. Unilateral megalencephaly is associated with severe mental retardation and untreatable seizures.

DESTRUCTIVE CEREBRAL LESIONS

These lesions include hydranencephaly, porencephaly and schizencephaly. In *hydranencephaly*, there is absence of the cerebral hemispheres with preservation of the mid-brain and cerebellum. In *porencephaly*, there are cystic cavities within the brain that usually communicate with the ventricular system, the subarachnoid space or both. *Schizencephaly* is associated with clefts in the fetal brain connecting the lateral ventricles with the subarachnoid space.

Prevalence

Destructive cerebral lesions are found in about 1 per 10 000 births.

Etiology

Hydranencephaly is a sporadic abnormality that may result from widespread vascular occlusion in the distribution of the internal carotid arteries, prolonged severe hydrocephalus, or an overwhelming infection such as toxoplasmosis or cytomegalovirus. Porencephaly may be caused by infarction of the cerebral arteries or hemorrhage into the brain parenchyma. Schizencephaly may be a primary disorder of brain development or it may be due to bilateral occlusion of the middle cerebral arteries.

Diagnosis

Complete absence of echoes from the anterior and middle fossae distinguishes hydranencephaly from severe hydrocephalus in which a thin rim of remaining cortex and the mid-line echo can always be identified. In porencephaly, there are one or more cystic areas in the cerebral cortex, which usually communicates with the ventricle; the differential diagnosis is from intracranial cysts (arachnoid, glyo-ependymal), that are usually found either within the scissurae or in the mid-line and compress the brain. In schizencephaly, there are bilateral clefts extending from the lateral ventricles to the subarachnoid space. Schizencephaly is usually associated with absence of the cavum septum pellucidum.

Prognosis

Hydranencephaly is usually incompatible with survival beyond early infancy. The prognosis in porencephaly is related to the size and location of the lesion and, although there is increased risk of impaired neurodevelopment in some cases, development is normal. Schizencephaly is associated with severe neurodevelopmental delay and seizures.

CHOROID PLEXUS CYSTS

These cysts, which are usually bilateral, are in the choroid plexuses of the lateral cerebral ventricles.

Prevalence

Choroid plexus cysts are found in about 2% of fetuses at 20 weeks of gestation, but in more than 90% of cases they resolve by 26 weeks.

Etiology

The choroid plexus is easily visualized from 10 weeks of gestation when it occupies almost the entire hemisphere. Thereafter and until 26 weeks, there is a rapid decrease in both the size of the choroid plexus and of the lateral cerebral ventricle in relation to the hemisphere. Choroid plexus cysts contain cerebrospinal fluid and cellular debris.

Diagnosis

The diagnosis is made by the presence of single or multiple cystic areas (greater than 2 mm in diameter) in one or both choroid plexuses.

Prognosis

They are usually of no pathological significance, but they are associated with an increased risk for trisomy 18 and possibly trisomy 21. In the absence of other markers of trisomy 18, the maternal age-related risk is increased by a factor of 1.5 (see Appendix I).

VEIN OF GALEN ANEURYSM

This is a mid-line aneurysmal dilatation of the vein of Galen due to an arteriovenous malformation with major hemodynamic disturbances.

Prevalence

Vein of Galen aneurysm is a very rare abnormality.

Etiology

Vein of Galen aneurysm is a sporadic abnormality.

Diagnosis

The diagnosis is made by the demonstration of a supratentorial mid-line translucent elongated cyst. Color Doppler demonstrates active arteriovenous flow within the cyst. There may be associated evidence of high-output heart failure.

Prognosis

In the neonatal period, about 50% of the infants present with heart failure and the rest are asymptomatic. In later life, hydrocephalus and intracranial hemorrhage may develop. Good results can be achieved by catheterization and embolization of the malformation.

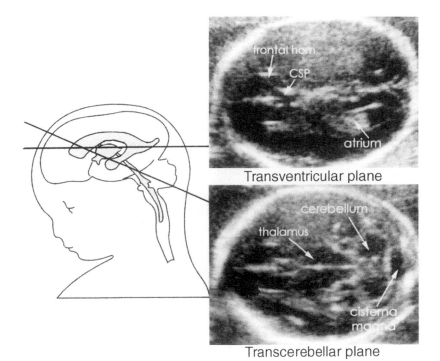

Figure 2 Normal brain

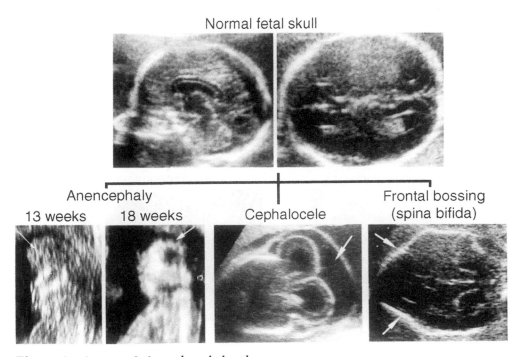

Figure 3 Anencephaly and cephalocele

Normal spine

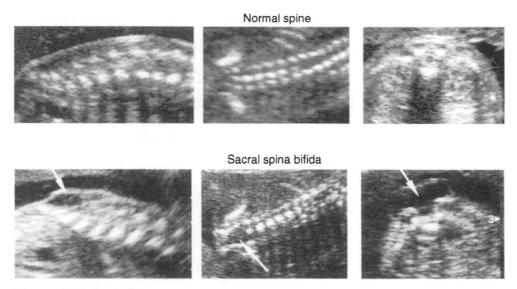

Sacral spina bifida

Figure 4 Spina bifida

Normal transventricular view

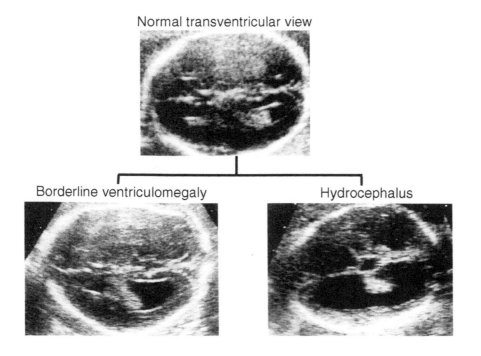

Borderline ventriculomegaly

Hydrocephalus

Figure 5 Ventriculomegaly and hydrocephalus

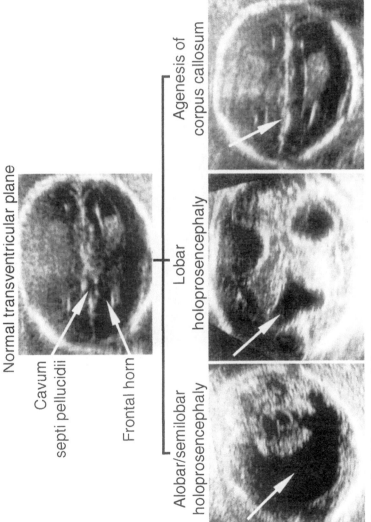

Normal transventricular plane

Cavum septi pellucidii

Frontal horn

Agenesis of corpus callosum

Lobar holoprosencephaly

Alobar/semilobar holoprosencephaly

Figure 6 Holoprosencephaly

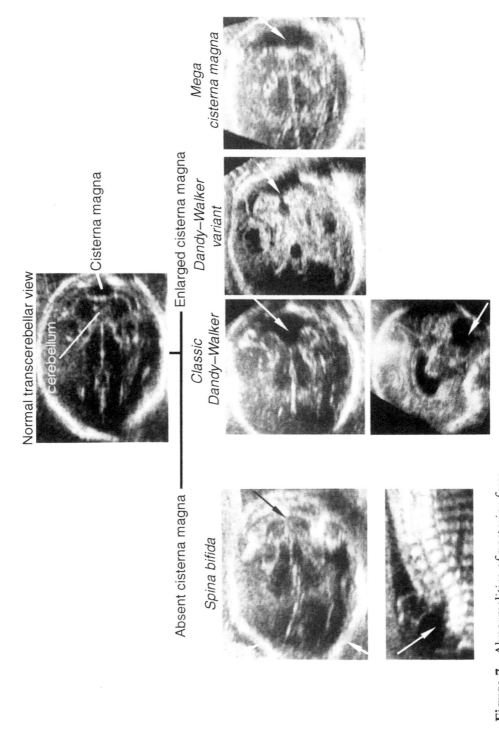

Figure 7 Abnormalities of posterior fossa

3

Face

NORMAL SONOGRAPHIC ANATOMY

The forehead, orbits, nose, lips and ears can be consistently identified from 12 weeks of gestation. Sagittal, transverse and coronal planes are all useful for the evaluation of normal and abnormal anatomy. A mid-sagittal plane allows visualization of the fetal profile (see Figure 8, p. 23), whereas the ears are visualized in parasagittal scans tangential to the calvarium. A series of transverse scans from the top of the head moving caudally allows examination of the forehead, nasal bridge, orbits, nose, upper lip and anterior palate, the tongue within the oral cavity, lower lip and mandible. The presence and size of the eyes are assessed subjectively, but, in cases of suspected defects, measurement of the internal and external orbital diameters may be necessary. The internal orbital diameter is approximately one-third of the external orbital diameter. The coronal planes are probably the most important ones in the evaluation of the integrity of facial anatomy (see Figure 9, p. 24). Orbits, eyelids, nose and lips are well visualized. The tip of the nose, the alae nasi, and the columna are seen above the upper lip. The nostrils typically appear as two small anechoic areas. There is a close relation between the development of the mid-line facial structures (forehead, nose, interorbital structures and upper lip) and the differentiation process of the forebrain. Therefore, mid-line defects of the face are frequently associated with cerebral anomalies, mainly holoprosencephaly.

ORBITAL DEFECTS

Hypertelorism (euryopia)

In early development, the eyes are placed laterally in the primitive face in a fashion similar to that of lower animals with panoramic vision. As gestation progresses, they migrate toward the mid-line, creating favorable conditions for the development of stereoscopic vision. Hypertelorism is an increased interorbital distance and this can be either an isolated finding or associated with many clinical syndromes or malformations. The most common syndromes with hypertelorism are the median cleft syndrome (hypertelorism, median cleft lip with or without a median cleft of the hard palate and nose, and cranium bifidum occultum), craniosynostoses (including Apert, Crouzon, and Carpenter syndromes), agenesis of the corpus callosum and anterior encephaloceles. Hypertelorism *per se* results only in cosmetic problems and possible impairment of stereoscopic binocular vision. For severe cases, a number of operative procedures, such as canthoplasty, orbitoplasty, surgical positioning of the eyebrows, and rhinoplasty, have been proposed. The median cleft face syndrome is usually associated with normal intelligence and life span. However, there is a high likelihood of mental retardation when either extracephalic anomalies or an extreme degree of hypertelorism are found. The severity of the cosmetic disturbance should not be underestimated, because this syndrome may be associated with extremely grotesque features.

Hypotelorism (stenopia)

Hypotelorism (decreased interorbital distance) is almost always found in association with other severe anomalies, such as holoprosencephaly, trigonocephaly, microcephaly, Meckel syndrome, and chromosomal abnormalities. The prognosis, which depends on the associated anomalies, is usually very poor.

Microphthalmia / anophthalmia

Microphthalmia is defined as a decreased size of the eyeball and anophthalmia refers to the absence of the eye; however, the term anophthalmia should be reserved for the pathologist, who must demonstrate not only absence of the eye but also of optic nerves, chiasma, and tracts. Microphthalmia/anophthalmia, which is either unilateral or bilateral, is usually associated with one of about 25 genetic syndromes. In Goldenhar syndrome (found in about 1 per 5000 births), there is unilateral anophthalmia, together with ear and facial abnormalities. Prenatal diagnosis is based on the demonstration of decreased ocular diameter, and careful examination of the intraorbital anatomy is indicated to identify lens, pupil and optic nerve. Congenital microphthalmia is frequently associated with visual disorders and with other anomalies.

Dacrocystocele

Congenital obstruction of the nasolacrimal duct results in cystic dilatation of the proximal part of the duct. Dacrocystocele has been identified prenatally as a hypoechogenic mass inferior to the globe. The differential diagnosis includes anterior encephaloceles (they are often associated with intracranial abnormalities such as hydrocephalus), hemangiomas (they are usually solid or multiseptated), and dermoid cysts (these are usually located superolaterally). Postnatally, dacrocystoceles resolve spontaneously in about 90% of cases within the first 6 months of life.

FACIAL CLEFT

This term refers to a wide spectrum of clefting defects (unilateral, bilateral and, less commonly, mid-line), usually involving the upper lip, the palate, or both. Cleft palate without cleft lip is a distinct disorder. Facial clefts encompass a broad spectrum of severity, ranging from minimal defects, such as a bifid uvula, linear indentation of the lip, or submucous cleft of the soft palate, to large deep defects of the facial bones and soft tissues. The typical cleft lip will appear as a linear defect extending from one side of the lip into the nostril. Cleft palate associated with cleft lip may extend through the alveolar ridge and hard palate, reaching the floor of the nasal cavity or even the floor of the orbit. Isolated cleft palate may include defects of the hard palate, the soft palate, or both. Both cleft lip and palate are unilateral in about 75% of cases and the left side is more often involved than the right side.

Prevalence

Facial clefting is found in about 1 per 800 births. In about 50% of cases, both the lip and palate are defective, in 25% only the lip and in 25% only the palate is involved.

Etiology

The face is formed by the fusion of four outgrowths of mesenchyme (frontonasal, mandibular and paired maxillary swellings) and facial clefting is caused by failure of fusion of these swellings. Cleft lip, with or without cleft palate, is usually (more than 80% of cases) an isolated condition, but, in 20% of cases, it is associated with one of more than 100 genetic syndromes. Isolated cleft palate is a different condition and it is more commonly associated with any one of more than 200 genetic syndromes. All forms of inheritance have been described, including autosomal dominant, autosomal recessive, X-linked dominant and X-linked recessive. Associated anomalies are found in about 50% of patients with isolated cleft palate and in about 15% of those with cleft lip and palate. Chromosomal abnormalities (mainly trisomies 13 and 18) are found in 1–2% of cases, and exposure to teratogens (such as antiepileptic drugs) in about 5% of cases. Recurrences are type-specific; if the index case has cleft lip and palate, there is no increased risk for isolated cleft palate, and vice versa. Median cleft lip, which accounts for about 0.5% of all cases of cleft lip, is usually associated with holoprosencephaly or the oral–facial–digital syndrome.

Diagnosis

The sonographic diagnosis of cleft and palate depends on demonstration of a groove extending from one of the nostrils inside the lip and possibly the alveolar ridge. Both transverse and coronal planes can be used. The diagnosis of isolated cleft palate is difficult and, in cases at risk for Mendelian syndromes, fetoscopy may be necessary.

Prognosis

Minimal defects, such as linear indentations of the lips or submucosal cleft of the soft palate, may not require surgical correction. Larger defects cause cosmetic, swallowing and respiratory problems. Recent advances in surgical techniques have produced good cosmetic and functional results. However, prognosis depends primarily on the presence and type of associated anomalies.

MICROGNATHIA

Micrognathia is characterized by mandibular hypoplasia causing a receding chin.

Prevalence

Micrognathia is found in about 1 per 1000 births.

Etiology

Micrognathia is usually associated with genetic syndromes (such as Treacher Collins, Robin and Robert syndromes), chromosomal abnormalities (mainly trisomy 18 and triploidy) and teratogenic drugs (such as methotrexate). The Robin anomalad (severe micrognathia, glossoptosis and a posterior cleft palate or an arched palate) may be a sporadic isolated finding (in about 40% of cases) or it may be associated with other anomalies or with recognized genetic and non-genetic syndromes. Otocephaly is a rare, lethal, sporadic abnormality characterized by severe hypoplasia of the mandible (agnathia) and severe mid-line defects, including holoprosencephaly, anterior encephalocele, cyclopia, aglossia, microstomia, and mid-facial location of the ears ('ear-head').

Diagnosis

Micrognathia is a subjective finding in the mid-sagittal view of the face and is characterized by a prominent upper lip and receding chin. The diagnosis can be confirmed by the demonstration of a short mandible. Severe micrognathia is associated with polyhydramnios, possibly because of the glossoptosis preventing swallowing.

Prognosis

This depends on the presence of associated anomalies. Severe micrognathia can be a neonatal emergency due to airway obstruction by the tongue in the small oral cavity. If prenatal diagnosis is made, a pediatrician should be present in the delivery room and be prepared to intubate the infant. Otocephaly is lethal.

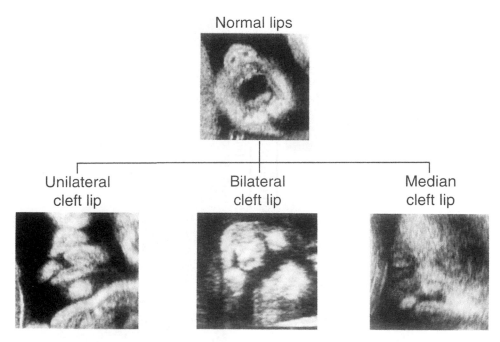

Figure 8 Facial cleft

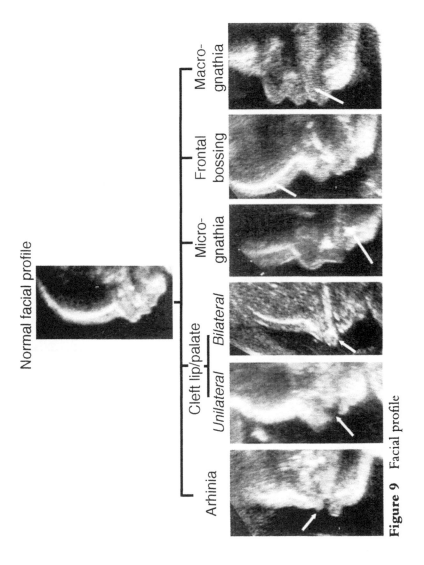

Figure 9 Facial profile

4

Cardiovascular system

Philippe Jeanty and Gianluigi Pilu

Abnormalities of the heart and great arteries are the most common congenital abnormalities. In general, about half are either lethal or require surgery and half are asymptomatic. The first two groups are referred to as major.

Prevalence

Cardiovascular abnormalities are found in 5–10 per 1000 live births and in about 30 per 1000 stillbirths.

Etiology

The etiology of heart defects is heterogeneous and probably depends on the interplay of multiple genetic and environmental factors, including maternal diabetes mellitus or collagen disease, exposure to drugs such as lithium, and viral infections such as rubella. Specific mutant gene defects and chromosomal abnormalities account for less than 5% of the patients. Heart defects are found in more than 90% of fetuses with trisomy 18 or 13, 50% of those with trisomy 21, and 40% of those with Turner syndrome, deletions or partial trisomies involving a variety of chromosomes.

Recurrence

When a previous sibling has had a congenital heart defect, in the absence of a known genetic syndrome, the risk of recurrence is about 2%, and with two affected siblings the risk is 10%. When the father is affected, the risk for the offspring is about 2% and if the mother is affected the risk is about 10%.

Reliability of prenatal diagnosis

Echocardiography has been successfully applied to the prenatal assessment of fetal cardiac function and structure, and has led to the diagnosis of most cardiac abnormalities. Studies from specialist centers report the diagnosis of about 90% of defects.

25

However, the majority of such studies refer to the prenatal diagnosis of moderate to major defects in high-risk populations.

Screening for cardiac abnormalities

The main challenge in prenatal diagnosis is to identify the high-risk group for referral to specialist centers. The indications include congenital cardiac defects in one of the parents or previous pregnancies, maternal diabetes mellitus or injestion of teratogenic drugs. However, more than 90% of fetuses with cardiac defects are from families without such risk factors. A higher sensitivity is achieved by examination of the four-chamber view of the heart at the routine 20-week scan; screening studies have reported the detection of about 30% of major cardiac defects. Recent evidence suggests that a higher sensitivity (more than 50%) can be achieved by referral for specialist echocardiography of patients with increased nuchal translucency at 10–14 weeks.

ASSESSMENT OF THE FETAL HEART

Real-time two-dimensional evaluation

The heart can be observed in an infinity of planes, but a few sections are the basis on which most of the diagnoses are made. These planes include the four-chamber, left and right chambers and great vessel views. Although it is convenient to refer to these standardized views for descriptive purposes, in practice it may be difficult to reproduce these exact sections, and the operator should be familiar with small variations of these planes.

Complex cardiac anomalies are frequently associated with an abnormal disposition of the heart and extracardiac viscera. Fetal echocardiography should always include an assessment of topographic anatomy of the abdomen and chest. The left and right sides are assessed by determining the relative position of the head and spine. The visceral situs is then assessed by demonstrating the relative position of the stomach, hepatic vessels, abdominal aorta and inferior vena cava.

A transverse section of the thorax reveals the four-chamber view of the fetal heart (see Figure 10, p. 49). The heart occupies approximately one-third of the thorax, and, in this view, the normal ventricles, atria, atrioventricular valves, ventricular and atrial septae, foramen ovale flap and pulmonary venous connections can be identified. The thicknesses of the interventricular septum and of the free ventricular walls are the same. The heart is not mid-line but shifted to the left side of the chest. The axis of the interventricular septum is about 45–20° to the left of the anteroposterior axis of the fetus. The interatrial septum is open at the level of the *foramen ovale*. The foramen ovale flap is visible in the left atrium, beating toward the left side. The insertion of the tricuspid valve along the interventricular septum is more apical than the insertion of the mitral valve. The confluence of the pulmonary veins into the left atrium serves to identify it as such. About 90% of ultrasonographically detectable fetal cardiac defects demonstrate some abnormalities in this view.

Evaluation of the cardiac outflow tracts can be difficult, but it is important to attempt such an examination because this improves the detection rate of many abnormalities of the heart and great arteries. The outflow tracts and great arteries can be demonstrated by slight angulations of the transducer from the four-chamber view (see Figure 11, p. 50). By turning the transducer while keeping the left ventricle and the aorta in the same plane, one can obtain the left heart views, while the right heart views are obtained by moving the transducer craniad and tilting slightly in the direction of the left shoulder. The views of the left heart demonstrate the left ventricle and aortic outflow tract. The anterior wall of the aorta is in continuity with the interventricular septum. The views of the right heart demonstrate the right ventricle and the right ventricular outflow tract. The main pulmonary artery originates from the anterior ventricle and trifurcates into a large vessel, the ductus going into the descending aorta, and two small vessels, the pulmonary arteries

There are two arches in the fetus (aortic arch and curve of the ductus) and they should be distinguished. The brachiocephalic vessels originate from the aortic arch, while no vessels emanate from the ductus. Furthermore, the curve of the aortic arch is gentler than that of the ductus, which is slightly more angular. The cavae can be seen in a longitudinal view as they both enter the right atrium.

M-mode

Heart rate and rhythm are assessed subjectively. M-mode, which is not used routinely, is useful for the evaluation of abnormal cases. In M-mode ultrasound, one line of information only is continuously displayed; instead of a two-dimensional scan of the heart, a recording of the variations of echoes along a single line is produced. Thus, M-mode is of little help in the analysis of the morphology of the heart but is useful in assessing motions and rhythms. One simply 'drops' an M-mode line over one atrial and ventricular wall. This allows one to quantitate cardiac frequency, and to infer the atrio-ventricular sequence of contractions.

Pulsed wave and color Doppler

Color Doppler overlays a representation of flow velocity over a conventional gray-scale image. This allows a rapid recognition of the flow pattern. Color Doppler is useful to assess normal anatomy and physiology, valvular regurgitation or stenosis, shunting and the orientation of flows. Pulsed wave Doppler is used to analyze the *spectral shift* (to assess the resistance in a vessel), to obtain *flow velocities* (how the resistance affects the flow), and *flow predictions* (to estimate the perfusion). Pulsed Doppler ultrasound, in combination with two-dimensional and M-mode sonography, has proved useful in the evaluation of both fetal dysrhythmias and structural anomalies. Pulsed Doppler can be useful in the detection and assessment of the severity of valvar abnormalities (stenosis, insufficiency). Analysis of atrioventricular inflows, hepatic veins and inferior vena cava can also be used to assess cardiac rhythm.

ATRIAL SEPTAL DEFECTS

Most atrial septal defects involve either the *septum primum* (the portion of the atrial septum below the foramen ovale) or the *septum secundum* (the portion above the foramen ovale). *Primum* atrial septal defect is the simplest form of the atrioventricular septal defects (see below). *Secundum* atrial septal defects, which are the most common, are usually isolated, but may be related to other cardiac lesions (such as mitral, pulmonary, tricuspid or aortic atresia) and are occasionally found as part of syndromes (including Holt–Oram syndrome in which there is hypo-aplasia of the thumb and radius, triphalangeal thumb, abrachia, and phocomelia).

Prevalence

Secundum atrial septal defects, which represent about 10% of congenital heart defects, are found in about 1 per 3000 births.

Diagnosis

Although the *in utero* identification of secundum atrial septal defect has been reported, the diagnosis remains difficult because of the physiological presence of the foramen ovale and only unusually large defects can be recognized with certainty.

Prognosis

Atrial septal defects are not a cause of impairment of cardiac function *in utero*, as a large right-to-left shunt at the level of the atria is a physiological condition in the fetus. Most affected babies are asymptomatic, even in the neonatal period.

VENTRICULAR SEPTAL DEFECTS

Defects in the ventricular septum are either isolated (about 50%) or they are part of a complex heart defect. They are classified into perimembranous, inlet, trabecular or outlet defects, depending on their location on the septum. *Perimembranous* defects (80%) involve the membranous septum below the aortic valve, but also extend in variable degrees into the adjacent portion of the septum. The *inlet* defects are on the inflow tract of the right ventricle and thus affect the implantation of the septal chordae of the tricuspid valve. The *trabecular* defects occur in the muscular portion of the septum, and the *outlet* defects are in the infundibular portion of the right ventricle.

Prevalence

Ventricular septal defects, which represent 30% of all congenital heart defects, are found in about 2 per 1000 births.

Diagnosis

Echocardiographic diagnosis depends on the demonstration of a dropout of echoes in the ventricular septum. Since most ventricular septal defects are perimembranous and subaortic, a detailed view of the left outflow tract is the best picture to image them. While evaluating the ventricular septum in search of defects, multiple views should be used. Perimembranous defects will be best demonstrated by the four-chamber view. Muscular defects (which are difficult to detect) are best searched for in the short-axis view by trying to demonstrate a connection between the two ventricles. Overall, small isolated ventricular septal defects are difficult to detect prenatally, and both false-positive and false-negative diagnoses have been made. Because of their position, outlet defects are not only beneath the aortic valve but also the pulmonary valve. They are the type associated with tetralogy of Fallot. Trabecular defects have not been detected by prenatal ultrasound because they are usually composed of small orifices.

Prognosis

Ventricular septal defects are not associated with hemodynamic compromise *in utero* because the right and left ventricular pressures are believed to be equal. More than 90% of small defects close spontaneously within the first year of life. Large defects present with congestive heart failure at 2–8 weeks of life and require medical treatment (digoxin and diuretics). Rarely, very large defects, associated with massive left-to-right shunt, can be associated with congestive heart failure soon after birth. If medical treatment fails, surgical closure is undertaken; survival from surgery is more than 90% and survivors have a normal life expectancy and normal exercise tolerance.

ATRIOVENTRICULAR SEPTAL DEFECTS

The ontogenesis of the apical portion of the atrial septum, of the basal portion of the interventricular septum and of the atrioventricular valves depends on development of mesenchymal masses (endocardial cushions). Abnormal development of these structures is commonly referred to as endocardial cushion defects, atrioventricular canal or atrioventricular septal defects. In the complete form, *persistent common atrioventricular canal*, the tricuspid and mitral valve are fused in a large, single atrioventricular valve that opens above and bridges the two ventricles. In the complete form of atrioventricular canal, the common atrioventricular valve may be incompetent, and systolic blood regurgitation from the ventricles to the atria may give rise to congestive heart failure.

Prevalence

Atrioventricular septal defects, which represent about 7% of all congenital heart defects, are found in about 1 per 3000 births.

Diagnosis

Antenatal echocardiographic diagnosis of complete atrioventricular septal defects is usually easy. An obvious deficiency of the central core structures of the heart is present. Color Doppler ultrasound can be useful, in that it facilitates the visualization of the central opening of the single atrioventricular valve. The atria may be dilated as a consequence of atrioventricular insufficiency. In such cases, color and pulsed Doppler ultrasound allow one to identify the regurgitant jet. The incomplete forms are more difficult to recognize. A useful hint is the demonstration that the tricuspid and mitral valves attach at the same level at the crest of the septum. This apical displacement of the mitral valve elongates the left ventricular outflow tract. The atrial septal defect is of the ostium primum type (since the septum secundum is not affected) and thus is close to the crest of the interventricular septum.

Prognosis

Atrioventricular septal defects will usually be encountered either in fetuses with chromosomal aberrations (50% of cases are associated with aneuploidy, 60% being trisomy 21, 25% trisomy 18) or in fetuses with cardiosplenic syndromes. In the former cases, an atrioventricular septal defect is frequently found in association with extracardiac anomalies. In the latter cases, multiple cardiac anomalies and abnormal disposition of the abdominal organs are almost the rule.

Atrioventricular septal defects do not impair the fetal circulation *per se*. However, the presence of atrioventricular valve insufficiency may lead to intrauterine heart failure. The prognosis of atrioventricular septal defects is poor when detected *in utero*, probably because of the high frequency of associated anomalies in antenatal series. About 50% of untreated infants die within the 1st year of life from heart failure, arrhythmias and pulmonary hypertension due to right-to-left shunting (Eisenmenger syndrome). Survival after surgical closure (which is usually carried out in the 6th month of life) is more than 90%, but in about 10% of patients a second operation for atrioventricular valve repair or replacement is necessary. Long-term prognosis is good.

CARDIOSPLENIC SYNDROMES

In cardiosplenic syndromes, also referred to as heterotaxy, the fetus is made of either two left or two right sides. Other terms commonly used include left or right isomerism, asplenia and polysplenia. Unpaired organs (liver, stomach and spleen) may be absent, mid-line or duplicated. Because of left atrial isomerism (and thus absence of the right atrium, which is the normal location for the pacemaker) and abnormal atrioventricular junctions, atrioventricular blocks are very common.

Prevalence

Cardiosplenic syndromes, which represent about 2% of all congenital heart defects, are found in about 1 in 10 000 births.

Polysplenia

In polysplenia, the fetus has two left sides (one in normal position and the other as a mirror image); this is called left isomerism. Multiple small spleens (usually too small to be detected by antenatal ultrasound) are found posterior to the stomach. The liver is mid-line and symmetric, but the stomach and aorta can be on opposite sides. Cardiac anomalies are almost invariably present, including anomalous pulmonary venous return, atrioventricular canal, and obstructive lesions of the aortic valve. One typical and peculiar finding is the interruption of the inferior vena cava, with the lower portion of the body drained by the azygos vein.

Evaluation of the disposition of the abdominal organs is of special value for the sonographic diagnosis of fetal cardiosplenic syndromes. In normal fetuses, a transverse section of the abdomen demonstrates the aorta on the left side and the inferior vena cava on the right; the stomach is to the left and the portal sinus of the liver bends to the right, towards the gallbladder. In polysplenia, a typical finding is interruption of the inferior vena cava with azygous continuation (there is failure to visualize the inferior vena cava and a large venous vessel, the azygos vein, runs to the left and close to the spine and ascends into the upper thorax). Symmetry of the liver can be sonographically recognized *in utero* by the abnormal course of the portal circulation that does not display a clearly defined portal sinus bending to the right.

The heterogeneous cardiac anomalies found in association with polysplenia are usually easily seen, but a detailed diagnosis often poses a challenge; in particular, assessment of a connection between the pulmonary veins and the atrium (an element that has a major prognostic influence) can be extremely difficult. Associated anomalies include absence of the gallbladder, malrotation of the guts, duodenal atresia and hydrops.

Asplenia

In asplenia, the fetus has two right sides (right isomerism). As in polysplenia, evaluation of the disposition of the abdominal organs is a major clue to the diagnosis. The liver is generally mid-line and the stomach right- or left-sided. The aorta and cava are on the same side (either left or right) of the spine. The spleen cannot be seen and the stomach is found in close contact with the thoracic wall. Cardiac malformations are severe, with a tendency towards a single structure replacing normal paired structures, for example, single atrium, single atrioventricular valve, single ventricle and single great vessel, and are usually easily demonstrated.

Diagnosis

Cardiosplenic syndromes may be inferred by the abnormal disposition of the abdominal organs. The presence of complex cardiac abnormalities is almost the rule.

Prognosis

The outcome depends on the severity of cardiac anomalies, but it tends to be poor. Atrioventricular insufficiency and severe fetal bradycardia due to atrioventricular block may lead to intrauterine heart failure.

UNIVENTRICULAR HEART

This term defines a group of anomalies characterized by the presence of an atrioventricular junction that is entirely connected to only one chamber in the ventricular mass. Therefore, univentricular heart includes both those cases in which two atrial chambers are connected, by either two distinct atrioventricular valves or by a common one, to a main ventricular chamber (double-inlet single ventricle), as well as those cases in which, because of the absence of one atrioventricular connection (tricuspid or mitral atresia), one of the ventricular chambers is either rudimentary or absent.

Prevalence

Univentricular heart is rare; it represents about 1.5% of all congenital cardiac defects.

Diagnosis

In double-outlet single ventricle, two separate atrioventricular valves are seen opening into a single ventricular cavity, without evidence of the interventricular septum. In mitral/tricuspid atresia, there is only one atrioventricular valve connected to a main ventricular chamber. A small rudimentary ventricular chamber, lacking an atrioventricular connection, is a frequent but not constant finding. Demonstration of two patent great arteries arising from the ventricle allows a differential diagnosis from hypoplastic ventricles (hypoplastic left heart syndrome, pulmonary atresia with intact ventricular septum).

Prognosis

Surgical treatment (the Fontan procedure) involves separation of the systemic circulations by anastomosing the superior and inferior vena cava directly to the pulmonary artery. The survivors from this procedure often have long-term complications, including arrhythmias, thrombus formation and protein-losing enteropathy. The 5-year survival is about 70%.

AORTIC STENOSIS

Aortic stenosis is commonly divided into supravalvar, valvar and subaortic forms. Supravalvar aortic stenosis can be due to one of three anatomic defects: a membrane (usually placed above the sinuses of Valsalva), a localized narrowing of the ascending aorta (hour-glass deformity) or a diffuse narrowing involving the aortic arch and branching arteries (tubular variety). The valvar form of aortic stenosis can be due to dysplastic, thickened aortic cusps or fusion of the commissure between the cusps. The subaortic forms include a fixed type, representing the consequence of a fibrous or fibromuscular obstruction, and a dynamic type, which is due to a thickened ventricular septum obstructing the outflow tract of the left ventricle. The latter is also known as asymmetric septal hypertrophy or idiopathic hypertrophic subaortic stenosis. A transient form of dynamic obstruction of the left outflow tract is seen in infants of diabetic mothers, and is probably the consequence of fetal hyperglycemia and hyperinsulinemia.

Prevalence

Aortic stenosis, which represents 3% of all congenital heart defects, is found in about 1 per 7000 births.

Diagnosis

Most cases of mild to moderate aortic stenosis are probably not amenable to early prenatal diagnosis. Severe valvar aortic stenosis of the fetus is usually associated with a hypertrophic left ventricle. Within the ascending aorta (that can be small or enlarged), pulsed Doppler demonstrates increased peak velocity (usually in excess of 1 m/s). At the color Doppler examination, high velocity and turbulence result in aliasing, with a mosaic of colors. Severe aortic stenosis may result in atrioventricular valve insufficiency and intrauterine heart failure. Asymmetric septal hypertrophy and hypertrophic cardiomyopathy of fetuses of diabetic mothers, resulting in subaortic stenosis, has been occasionally diagnosed by demonstrating an unusual thickness of the ventricular septum. We are not aware of cases of supravalvular aortic stenosis detected *in utero*.

Prognosis

Depending upon the severity of the aortic stenosis, the association of left ventricular pressure overload and subendocardial ischemia, due to decrease in coronary perfusion, may lead to intrauterine impairment of cardiac function. Subvalvular and subaortic forms are not generally manifested in the neonatal period. Conversely, the valvar type can be a cause of congestive heart failure in the newborn and fetus as well. Although there is concern that cases seen in early gestation may progress in severity, the lesion usually remains stable. The neonatal outcome depends on the severity of obstruction. If the left ventricular function is adequate, balloon valvoplasty is carried out in the neonatal period and, in about 50% of cases, surgery is necessary within the first 10 years of life because of aortic insufficiency or residual stenosis. If left ventricular function is inadequate, a Norwood-type of repair is necessary (see hypoplastic left heart).

Fetal therapy

Antenatal transventricular balloon valvuloplasty has been attempted in a handful of cases but the results are uncertain.

COARCTATION AND TUBULAR HYPOPLASIA OF THE AORTA

Coarctation is a localized narrowing of the juxtaductal arch, most commonly between the left subclavian artery and the ductus. Cardiac anomalies are present in 90% of the cases and include aortic stenosis and insufficiency, ventricular septal defect, atrial septal defect, transposition of the great arteries, truncus and double-outlet right ventricle. Non-cardiac anomalies include diaphragmatic hernia, Turner syndrome but not Noonan syndrome.

Diagnosis

Coarctation may be a postnatal event, and this limits prenatal diagnosis in many cases. It should be suspected when the right ventricle is enlarged (right ventricle to left ventricle ratio of more than 1.3). Narrowing of the isthmus, or the presence of a shelf, are often difficult to demonstrate because, in the fetus, aortic arch and ductal arch are close and are difficult to distinguish. In most cases, coarctation can only be suspected *in utero* and a certain diagnosis must be delayed until after birth.

Prognosis

Critical coarctation is fatal in the neonatal period after closure of the ductus and therefore prostaglandin therapy is necessary to maintain a patent ductus. Surgery (which involves excision of the coarcted segment and end-to-end anastomosis) is associated with a mortality of about 10% and the incidence of re-stenosis in survivors (requiring further surgical repair) is about 15%.

INTERRUPTED AORTIC ARCH

The interruption of the aortic arch can be complete or there may be an atretic fibrous segment between the arch and the descending aorta. It may be isolated or associated with intracardiac lesions that cause obstruction to the blood flow from the left heart (aortic stenosis, aortic atresia, malaligned ventricular septal defects). Associated extracardiac anomalies are frequent and include DiGeorge syndrome (association of thymic aplasia, type B interruption and hypoplastic mandible), holoprosencephaly, cleft lip/palate, esophageal atresia, duplicated stomach, diaphragmatic hernia, horseshoe kidneys, bilateral renal agenesis, oligodactyly, claw hand and syrenomelia.

Diagnosis

Interrupted aortic arch should always be considered when intracardiac lesions diverting blood flow from the left to the right heart are encountered (aortic stenosis and atresia in particular). Isolated interruption of the aortic arch is often encountered with enlargement of the right ventricle (right ventricle to left ventricle ratio of more than 1.3). As the sonographic access to the arch is difficult, the diagnosis is not always possible. The characteristic finding of an ascending aorta more vertical than usually, and the impossibility to demonstrate a connection with the descending aorta, suggest the diagnosis.

Prognosis

The median age at death for unoperated infants is 4 days. The initial treatment is the same as for any anomalies in which the perfusion is ductus-dependent: prostaglandin E_1. Recent reports suggest an overall late survival of more than 70% after surgery.

HYPOPLASTIC LEFT HEART SYNDROME

This is a spectrum of anomalies characterized by a very small left ventricle with mitral and/or aortic atresia or hypoplasia. Blood flow to the head and neck vessels and coronary artery is supplied in a retrograde manner via the ductus arteriosus.

Diagnosis

Prenatal echocardiographic diagnosis of the syndrome depends on the demonstration of a diminutive left ventricle and ascending aorta. In most cases, the ultrasound appearance is self-explanatory, and the diagnosis an easy one. There is, however, a broad spectrum of hypoplasia of the left ventricle and, in some cases, the ventricular cavity is almost normal in size. As the four-chamber view is almost normal, we anticipate that these cases will be certainly missed in most routine surveys of fetal anatomy. At a closer scrutiny, however, the movement of the mitral valve appears severely impaired to non-existent, ventricular contractility is obviously decreased, and the ventricle often displays an internal echogenic lining that is probably due to endocardial fibroelastosis. The definitive diagnosis of the syndrome depends on the demonstration of hypoplasia of the ascending aorta and atresia of the aortic valve. Color flow mapping is an extremely useful adjunct to the real-time examination, in that it allows the demonstration of retrograde blood flow within the ascending aorta and aortic arch.

Prognosis

Hypoplastic left heart is well tolerated *in utero*. The patency of the ductus arteriosus allows adequate perfusion of the head and neck vessels. Intrauterine growth may be normal, and the onset of symptoms most frequently occurs after birth. The prognosis for infants with hypoplastic left heart syndrome is extremely poor and this lesion is responsible for 25% of cardiac deaths in the 1st week of life. Almost all affected infants die within 6 weeks if they are not treated. In the neonatal period, prostaglandin therapy is given to maintain ductal patency, but still congestive heart failure develops within 24 h of life. Options for surgery include cardiac transplantation in the neonatal period (with an 80% 5-year survival) and the three-staged Norwood repair. Stage 1 involves anastomosis of the pulmonary artery to the aortic arch for systemic outflow, placement of systemic-to-pulmonary arterial shunt to provide pulmonary blood flow, and arterial septectomy to ensure unobstructed pulmonary venous return; the mortality from the procedure is about 30%. Stage 2 (which is usually carried out in the 6th month of life) involves anastomosis of the superior vena cava to the pulmonary arteries. The overall 2-year survival with the Norwood repair is about 50%, but more than 50% of survivors have neurodevelopmental delay.

PULMONARY STENOSIS AND PULMONARY ATRESIA

Prevalence

Pulmonary stenosis is found in about 1 per 2000 births. Pulmonary atresia is rare, and is found in less than 1 per 10 000 births.

Diagnosis

The most common form of pulmonary stenosis is the valvar type, due to the fusion of the pulmonary leaflets. Hemodynamics are altered in proportion to the degree of the stenosis. The work of the right ventricle is increased, as well as the pressure, leading to hypertrophy of the ventricular walls. The same considerations formulated for the prenatal diagnosis of aortic stenosis are valid for pulmonary stenosis as well. A handful of cases recognized *in utero* have been reported in the literature thus far, mostly severe types with enlargement of the right ventricle and/or post-stenotic enlargement or hypoplasia of the pulmonary artery.

Pulmonary atresia with intact ventricular septum (PA:IVS) in infants is usually associated with an hypoplastic right ventricle. However, cases with enlarged right ventricle and atrium have been described with unusual frequency in prenatal series. Although these series are small, it is possible that the discrepancy with the pediatric literature is due to the very high perinatal loss rate that is found in 'dilated' cases. Enlargement of the ventricle and atrium is probably the consequence of tricuspid insufficiency. Prenatal diagnosis of PA:IVS relies on the demonstration of a small pulmonary artery with an atretic pulmonary valve. The considerations previously formulated for the diagnosis of hypoplastic left heart syndrome apply to PA:IVS as well.

Prognosis

Patients with mild stenosis are asymptomatic and there is no need for intervention. Patients with severe stenosis, right ventricular overload may result in congestive heart failure and require balloon valvoplasty in the neonatal period with excellent survival and normal long-term prognosis. Fetuses with pulmonary atresia and an enlarged right heart have a very high degree of perinatal mortality. Infants with right ventricular hypoplasia require biventricular surgical repair and the mortality is about 40%.

CONOTRUNCAL MALFORMATIONS

Conotruncal malformations are a heterogeneous group of defects that involve two different segments of the heart: the conotruncus and the ventricles. Conotruncal anomalies are relatively frequent. They account for 20–30% of all cardiac anomalies and are the leading cause of symptomatic cyanotic heart disease in the first year of life. Prenatal diagnosis is of interest for several reasons. Given the parallel model of fetal circulation, conotruncal anomalies are well tolerated *in utero*. The clinical presentation occurs usually hours to days after delivery, and is often severe, representing a true emergency and leading to considerable morbidity and mortality. Yet, these malformations have a good prognosis when promptly treated. Two ventricles of adequate size and two great vessels are commonly present, giving the premise for biventricular surgical correction. The outcome is indeed much more favorable than with most of the other cardiac defects that are detected antenatally. The first reports on prenatal echocardiography of conotruncal malformations date back from the beginning of the 1980s. Nevertheless, despite improvement in the technology of diagnostic ultrasound, the recognition of these anomalies remains difficult. The four-chamber view is frequently unremarkable in these cases. A specific diagnosis requires meticulous scanning and at times may represent a challenge even for experienced sonologists. Referral centers with special expertise in fetal echocardiography have indeed reported both false-positive and false-negative diagnoses.

TRANSPOSITION OF THE GREAT ARTERIES

Transposition of the great arteries is an abnormality in which the aorta arises entirely or in large part from the right ventricle and the pulmonary artery arises from the left ventricle. Associated cardiac lesions are present in about 50% of cases, including ventricular septal defects (which can occur anywhere in the ventricular septum), pulmonary stenosis, unbalanced ventricular size ('complex transpositions'), anomalies of the mitral valve, which can be straddling or overridding. There are three types of complete transposition: those with intact ventricular septum with or without pulmonary stenosis, those with ventricular septal defects and those with ventricular septal defect and pulmonary stenosis.

Prevalence

Transposition of the great arteries is found in about 1 per 5000 births.

Diagnosis

Complete transposition is probably one of the most difficult cardiac lesions to recognize *in utero*. In most cases, the four-chamber view is normal, and the cardiac cavities and the vessels have normal appearance. A clue to the diagnosis is the demonstration that the two great vessels do not cross but arise parallel from the base of the heart. The most useful echocardiographic view, however, is the left heart view, demonstrating that the vessel connected to the left ventricle has a posterior course and bifurcates into the two pulmonary arteries. Conversely, the vessel connected to the right ventricle has a long upward couse and gives rise to the brachiocephalic vessels. Difficulties may arise in the case of huge malalignment ventricular septal defect with overriding of the posterior semilunar root. This combination makes the differentiation with double-outlet right ventricle very difficult. Corrected transposition is characterized by a double discordance, at the atrioventricular and ventriculo-arterial level. The left atrium is connected to the right ventricle, which is in turn connected to the ascending aorta. Conversely, the right atrium is connected with the right ventricle, which is in turn connected to the ascending aorta. The derangement of the conduction tissue secondary to malalignment of the atrial and ventricular septa may result in dysrhythmias, namely complete atrioventricular block. For diagnostic purposes, the identification of the peculiar difference of ventricular morphology (moderator band, papillary muscles, insertion of the atrioventricular valves) has a prominent role. Demonstration that the pulmonary veins are connected to an atrium which is in turn connected with a ventricle that has the moderator band at the apex is an important clue, that is furthermore potentially identifiable even in a simple four-chamber view. Diagnosis requires meticolous scanning to assess carefully all cardiac connections, by using the same views described for the complete form. The presence of atrioventricular block increases the index of suspicion.

Prognosis

As anticipated from the parallel model of fetal circulation, complete transposition is uneventful *in utero*. After birth, survival depends on the amount and size of the mixing of the two otherwise independent circulations. Patients with transposition and an intact ventricular septum present shortly after birth with cyanosis and deteriorate rapidly. When a large ventricular septal defect is present, cyanosis can be mild. Clinical presentation may be delayed up to 2–4 weeks, and usually occurs with signs of congestive heart failure. When severe stenosis of the pulmonary artery is associated with a ventricular septal defect, symptoms are similar to patients with tetralogy of Fallot. The time and mode of clinical presentation with corrected transposition depend upon the concomitant cardiac defects.

Surgery (which involves arterial switch to establish anatomic and physiological correction) is usually carried out within the first 2 weeks of life. Operative mortality is about 10% and 10-year follow-up studies report normal function, but there is uncertainty if, in the long-term, such patients are at increased risk of atherosclerotic coronary disease. In cases with pulmonary stenosis and ventricular septal defect, balloon atrial septostomy may be necessary to ensure adequate oxygenation until definitive repair when the patient is older.

DOUBLE-OUTLET RIGHT VENTRICLE

In double-outlet right ventricle (DORV), most of the aorta and pulmonary valve arise completely or almost completely from the right ventricle. The relation between the two vessels may vary, ranging from a Fallot-like to a TGA-like situation (the Taussig–Bing anomaly). DORV is not a single malformation from a pathophysiological point of view. The term refers only to the position of the great vessels that is found in association with ventricular septal defects, tetralogy of Fallot, transposition, univentricular hearts. Pulmonary stenosis is very common in all types of DORV, but left outflow obstructions, from subaortic stenosis to coarctation and interruption of the aortic arch, can also be seen.

Prevalence

Double-outlet right ventricle is found in less than 1 per 10 000 births.

Diagnosis

Prenatal diagnosis of DORV can be reliably made in the fetus but differentiation from other conotruncal anomalies can be very difficult, especially with tetralogy of Fallot and transposition of the great arteries with ventricular septal defect. The main echocardiographic features include, first, alignment of the two vessels totally or predominantly from the right ventricle, and, second, the presence in most cases of bilateral coni (subaortic and subpulmonary). The hemodynamics are dependent upon the anatomic type of DORV and the associated anomalies. Since the fetal heart works as a common chamber where the blood is mixed and pumped, DORV is not associated with intrauterine heart failure. However, DORV, in contrast to other conotruncal malformations, is commonly associated with extracardiac anomalies and/or chromosomal defects.

Prognosis

Double-outlet right ventricle usually does not interfere with hemodynamics in fetal life. The early operative mortality is about 10%.

TETRALOGY OF FALLOT

The essential features of this malformation are, first, malalignment ventricular septal defect with anterior displacement of the infundibular septum associated with sub-pulmonary narrowing and overriding aortic root, and, second, demonstrable continuity betweeen the right outflow tract and the pulmonary trunk. In about 20% of cases, this continuity is lacking, leading to atresia of the pulmonary valve, a condition that is commonly referred to as pulmonary atresia with ventricular septal defect. Tetralogy of Fallot can be associated with other specific cardiac malformations, defining peculiar entities. These include atrioventricular septal defects (found in 4% of cases), and absence of the pulmonary valve (found in less than 2% of cases). Hypertrophy of the right ventricle, one of the classic elements of the tetrad, is always absent in the fetus, and only develops after birth.

Prevalence

Tetralogy of Fallot is found in about 1 per 3000 births.

Diagnosis

Echocardiographic diagnosis of tetralogy of Fallot relies on the demonstration of a ventricular septal defect in the outlet portion of the septum and an overriding aorta. There is an inverse relationship between the size of the ascending aorta and pulmonary artery, with a disproportion that is often striking. A large aortic root is indeed an important diagnostic clue. Doppler studies provide valuable information. The finding of increased peak velocities in the pulmonary artery corroborates the diagnosis of tetralogy of Fallot by suggesting obstruction to blood flow in the right outflow tract. Conversely, demonstration with color and/or pulsed Doppler that, in the pulmonary artery, there is either no forward flow or reverse flow allows a diagnosis of pulmonary atresia. Diagnostic problems arise at the extremes of the spectrum of tetralogy of Fallot. In cases with minor forms of right outflow obstruction and aortic overriding, differentiation from a simple ventricular septal defect can be difficult. In those cases in which the pulmonary artery is not imaged, a differential diagnosis between pulmonary atresia with ventricular septal defect and truncus arteriosus communis is similarly difficult. The sonographer should also be alerted to a frequent artifact that resembles overriding of the aorta. Incorrect orientation of the transducer may demonstrate apparent septo-aortic discontinuity in a normal fetus. The mechanism of the artifact is probably related to the angle of incidence of the sound beam. Careful visualization of the left outflow tract with different insonation angles, as well as the use of color Doppler and the research for the other elements of the tetralogy, should virtually eliminate this problem. Abnormal enlargement of the right ventricle, main pulmonary trunk and artery suggests absence of the pulmonary valve. Evaluation of other variables, such as multiple ventricular septal defects and coronary anomalies, would be valuable for a better prediction of surgical timing and operative prognosis. Unfortunately, these findings cannot be definitely recognized by prenatal echocardiography.

Prognosis

Cardiac failure is never seen in fetal life as well as postnatally. Even in cases of tight pulmonary stenosis or atresia, the wide ventricular septal defect provides adequate combined ventricular output, while the pulmonary vascular bed is supplied in a retrograde manner by the ductus. The only exception to this rule is represented by cases with an absent pulmonary valve that may result in massive regurgitation to the right ventricle and atrium. When severe pulmonary stenosis is present, cyanosis tends to develop immediately after birth. With lesser degrees of obstruction to pulmonary blood flow, the onset of cyanosis may not appear until later in the first year of life. When there is pulmonary atresia, rapid and severe deterioration follows ductal constriction. Survival after complete surgical repair (which is usually carried out in the 3rd month of life) is more than 90%, and about 80% of survivors have normal exercise tolerance.

TRUNCUS ARTERIOSUS COMMUNIS

Truncus arteriosus is characterized by a single arterial vessel that originates from the heart, overrides the ventricular septum and supplies the systemic, pulmonary and coronary circulations. The single arterial trunk is larger than the normal aortic root and is predominantly connected with the right ventricle in about 40% of cases, with the left ventricle in 20%, and is equally shared in 40%. The truncal valve may have one, two or three cusps and is rarely normal. It can be stenotic or, more frequently, insufficient. A malalignment ventricular septal defect, usually wide, is an essential part of the malformation. There are three types based on the morphology of the pulmonary artery. In type 1, the pulmonary arteries arise from the truncus within a short distance from the valve, as a main pulmonary trunk, which then bifurcates. In type 2, there is no main pulmonary trunk. In type 3, only one pulmonary artery (usually the right) originates from the truncus, while the other is supplied by a systemic collateral vessel from the descending aorta. Similar to the tetralogy of Fallot, and unlike the other conotruncal malformations, truncus is frequently (about 30%) associated with extracardiac malformations.

Prevalence

Truncus arteriosus is found in about 1 per 10 000 births.

Diagnosis

Truncus arteriosus can be reliably detected with fetal echocardiography. The main diagnostic criteria are, first, a single semilunar valve overrides the ventricular septal defect, and, second, there is direct continuity between one or two pulmonary arteries and the single arterial trunk. The semilunar valve is often thickened and moves abnormally. Doppler ultrasound is of value to assess incompetence of the truncal valve. A peculiar problem found in prenatal echocardiography is the demonstration of the absence of the pulmonary outflow tract and the concomitant failure to image the pulmonary arteries. In this situation, a differentiation between truncus and pulmonary atresia with ventricular septal defect may be impossible.

Prognosis

Similar to the other conotruncal anomalies, truncus arteriosus is not associated with alteration of fetal hemodynamics. Truncus arteriosus is frequently a neonatal emergency. These patients usually have unobstructed pulmonary blood flow and show signs of progressive congestive heart failure with the postnatal fall in pulmonary resistance. Many patients will present with cardiac failure in the first 1 or 2 weeks of life. Surgical repair (usually before the 6th month of life) involves closure of the ventricular septal defect and creation of a conduit connection between the right ventricle and the pulmonary arteries. Survival from surgery is about 90%, but the patients require repeated surgery for replacement of the conduit.

EBSTEIN'S ANOMALY AND TRICUSPID VALVE DYSPLASIA

Ebstein's anomaly results from a faulty implantation of the tricuspid valve. The posterior and septal leaflets are elongated and tethered below their normal level of attachment on the annulus or displaced apically, away from the annulus, down to the junction between the inlet and trabecular portion of the right ventricle. The anterior leaflet is normally inserted but deformed. The resulting configuration is that of a considerably enlarged right atrium at the expense of the right ventricle. The portion of the right ventricle that is ceded to the right atrium is called the *atrialized* inlet of the right ventricle. It has a thin wall that may even be membranous and is commonly dilated. The tricuspid valve is usually both incompetent and stenotic. Associated anomalies include atrial septal defect, pulmonary atresia, ventricular septal defect, and supraventricular tachycardia. Ebstein's anomaly may be associated with trisomies 13 and 21, Turner, Cornelia de Lange and Marfan syndromes. Maternal injestion of lithium has also been incriminated as a causal factor.

Diagnosis

The characteristic finding is that of a massively enlarged right atrium, a small right ventricle, and a small pulmonary artery. Doppler can be used to demonstrate regurgitation in the right atrium. About 25% of the cases have supraventricular tachycardia (from re-entrant impulse), atrial fibrillation or atrial flutter. Differential diagnosis from pulmonary atresia with intact ventricular septum and a regurgitant tricuspid valve or isolated tricuspid valve insufficiency is difficult and may be impossible antenatally.

Prognosis

Although the disease has a variable severity with some cases discovered only late in life, Ebstein's anomalies detected prenatally have a dismal prognosis, with essentially all patients dying. This probably reflects that the prenatal variety is more severe than the one detected in children or adults.

ECHOGENIC FOCI

Prevalence

Echogenic foci in the heart are found in about 4% of pregnancies and in 12% of fetuses with trisomy 21.

Etiology

Histological studies have shown these foci to be due to mineralization within a papillary muscle.

Diagnosis

Echogenic foci are detected in the four-chamber view of the heart. In about 95% of cases, they are located in the left ventricle and in 5% in the right ventricle; in 98% they are unilateral and 2% bilateral. Ventricular function is normal and the atrioventricular valves are competent.

Prognosis

Echogenic foci are usually of no pathological significance and, in more than 90% of cases, they resolve by the third trimester of pregnancy. However, they are sometimes associated with cardiac defects and chromosomal abnormalities. For isolated hyperechogenic foci, the risk for trisomy 21 may be three times the background maternal age- and gestation-related risk (see Appendix I).

CARDIAC DYSRHYTHMIAS: PREMATURE CONTRACTIONS

Ectopic heart beats are common but they are abnormal only when they occur at a frequency of more than one in ten beats. Premature contractions may be of atrial (much more common) or ventricular origin. Immaturity of the conducting system may be the origin. The diagnosis is made by passing an M-mode cursor through one atrium and one ventricle (see Figure 12, p. 51). Premature atrial contractions are spaced closer to the previous contraction than normally and may be transmitted to the ventricle or blocked. Premature ventricular contractions present in the same way but are not accompanied by an atrial contraction. Premature ventricular contractions are often followed by a *compensatory pause* due to the refractory state of the conduction system; the next conducted impulse arrives at twice the normal interval, and the continuity of the rhythm is not broken. Premature atrial contractions are usually followed by a *non-compensatory pause*; when the regular rhythm resumes, it is not synchronous with the rhythm before the extrasystole. The distance between the contraction that preceded the premature contraction and the one following it is not twice the distance between two normal contractions but a little shorter. Another approach to the sonographic diagnosis is to evaluate the waveforms obtained from the atrioventricular valves, hepatic vessels or inferior vena cava, which demonstrate pulsations corresponding to atrial and ventricular contractions.

Premature contractions are benign, tend to disappear spontaneously *in utero*, and only rarely persist after birth. It has been suggested that, in some cases, there may be progression to tachyarrhythmia, but the risk, if any, is certainly very small.

CARDIAC DYSRHYTHMIAS: TACHYARRHYTHMIAS

Tachyarrhythmias are classified according to the origin and the number of beats per minute. In the majority of cases, the abnormal electrical impulse originates from the atria. Atrial tachyarrhythmia includes *supraventricular tachycardia*, *atrial flutter* and *atrial fibrillation*. Since atrial rhythms greater than 240 beats/min are usually associated with varying degrees of atrioventricular block, the ventricular rate is usually reduced to 60–160 beats/min. Ventricular tachycardia has been occasionally encountered during fetal life. *Supraventricular tachycardia* is the most common form of tachyarrhythmia, and the ventricular response is 1 : 1. It is characterized by a heart rate of 200–300 beats/min. Supraventricular tachycardia may be due to an autonomous focus, in which case the rhythm is monotonous, or to a re-entry mechanism, in which case sudden conversion from an abnormal to a normal rhythm can be seen. Cardiac malformations are rare.

Atrial flutter is associated with a heart rate of 300–400 beats/min. The ventricular response is equal to or less than 2 : 1. Occasionally, atrioventricular block of high degree with ventricular bradycardia are seen. Structural anomalies are more common than in supraventricular tachycardia and include Ebstein's anomaly and pulmonary stenosis.

Atrial fibrillation is characterized by an atrial rate greater than 400 beats/min and completely irregular ventricular rhythm, with constant variation of the distance between systole. The atrial contractions are usually too small to be detected by M-mode. A combination of different atrial arrhythmias may coexist in the same fetus.

Ventricular tachycardias are rare, and have typically a ventricular frequency of 200 beats/min or less. Associated anomalies include atrial septal defect, atrial septal aneurysm, mitral anomalies, endocardial cushion defect, endocardial fibroelastosis, Ebstein's anomaly, cardiac tumors (rhabdomyoma), anomalies of the conduction system, Coxsackie B infection and cardiomyopathy. Tachycardia is commonly associated with hydrops, as a consequence of low cardiac output.

Diagnosis

The heart rate, atrial and ventricular, can be analyzed by either M-mode sonography of the cardiac chambers or pulsed Doppler evaluation of atrioventricular inflows, hepatic veins and inferior vena cava. A heart rate of about 240 beats/min with atrioventricular conduction of 1 : 1, is pathognomonic of supraventricular tachycardia. An atrial rate greater than 300 beats/min with an atrioventricular response of 1 : 2 or less indicates atrial flutter. A very fast atrial rate with irregular ventricular response is indicative of atrial fibrillation. A ventricular rate in the range of 200 beats/min with a normal atrial rate is suggestive of ventricular tachycardia.

Prognosis

Sustained tachycardia is associated with suboptimal ventricular filling and decreased cardiac output. These result in atrial overload and congestive failure. Fetuses with supraventricular tachycardia that occasionally convert to sinus rhythm can tolerate well the condition. Sustained tachycardias of greater than 200 beats/min frequently result in fetal hydrops. The combination of hydrops and dysrhythmia has a poor prognosis (mortality of 80%) independent of the nature of the tachycardia.

Fetal therapy

After 32 weeks of gestation, the fetus should be delivered and treated *ex utero*. Prenatal treatment is the standard of care for premature fetuses that have sustained tachycardias of more than 200 beats/min, particularly if there is associated hydrops and/or poly-hydramnios. The treatment depends on the type of tachycardia, and the aim is to either decrease the excitability or increase the conduction time to block a re-entrant mechanism. Although a vagual maneuver (such as simple compression of the cord) may sometimes suffice, the administration of antiarrhythmic drugs is often necessary. The drugs used include propranolol, verapamil, procainamide, quinidine, flecainide, amiodarone and adenosine; a combination of these drugs is also possible but the optimal approach remains uncertain. These drugs are usually administered to the mother but they can also be given directly to the fetus (intraperitoneally, intramuscularly in the thigh or intravascularly through the umbilical cord). The usual response to treatment is conversion to a normal rhythm, followed by shorter episodes of tachycardia that are more interspersed, and finally the presence of extrasystole alone. Fetuses with normal rhythm but persistent hydrops are still at risk of death. The survival rate of fetuses with tachyarrhythmias treated *in utero* is more than 90%.

CARDIAC DYSRHYTHMIAS: COMPLETE ATRIOVENTRICULAR BLOCK

In complete atrioventricular block, the atria beat at their own rhythm, and none of their impulses is transmitted to the ventricles. The ventricles have a slow rate (40–70 beats/min). In 50% of cases, structural anomalies are present (mostly left isomerism and corrected transposition of the great arteries). In the remaining cases, the condition is almost exclusively caused by the presence of maternal autoantibodies, anti-Ro (SS-a) or anti-La (SS-B). Most mothers are asymptomatic, but in a few cases connective tissue disease is present (lupus erythematosus, scleroderma, rheumatoid arthritis and Sjogren's syndrome). Fetuses with cardiac malformations have heart block starting from the first trimester. Atrioventricular block secondary to maternal auto-antibodies develops slowly throughout gestation; a normal cardiac rhythm may be found in the second trimester.

Atrial and ventricular contractions are identified by either M-mode or pulsed Doppler, as previously described. The prognosis depends on the presence of cardiac defects, the ventricular rate and the presence of hydrops; usually, fetuses with a ventricular rate greater than 55 beats/min have a normal intrauterine growth and do not develop heart failure. Conversely, hydrops is almost the rule for greater degrees of ventricular bradycardia. Intrauterine treatment by the administration of β-mimetic agents has been used (with the aim of increasing electric excitability of the myocardial cells and thus ventricular rate), but the results have been disappointing. Maternal administration of steroids (dexamethasone 8 mg/day) has been advocated for complete heart block secondary to maternal autoantibodies, but the value of this treatment remains, however, unproven. Invasive fetal cardiac pacing has been attempted but thus far there have been no survivors.

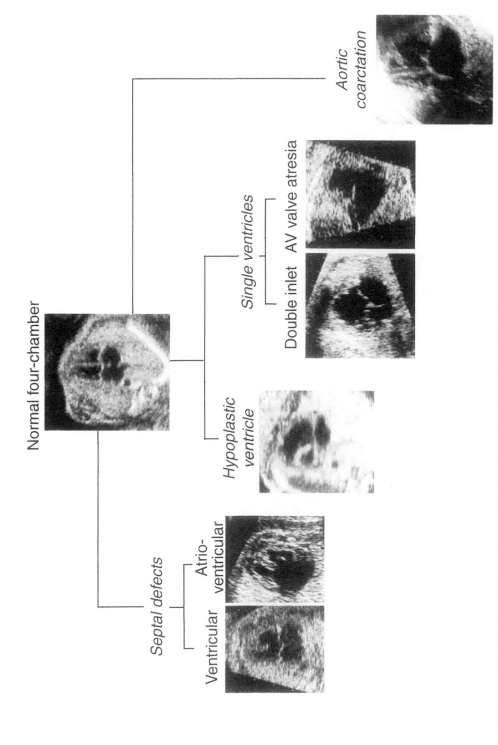

Figure 10 Cardiac defects detected in the four-chamber view of the heart

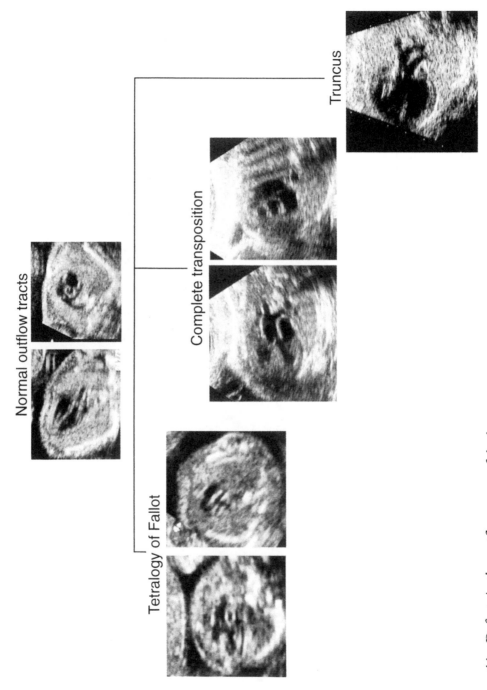

Figure 11 Defects in the outflow tracts of the heart

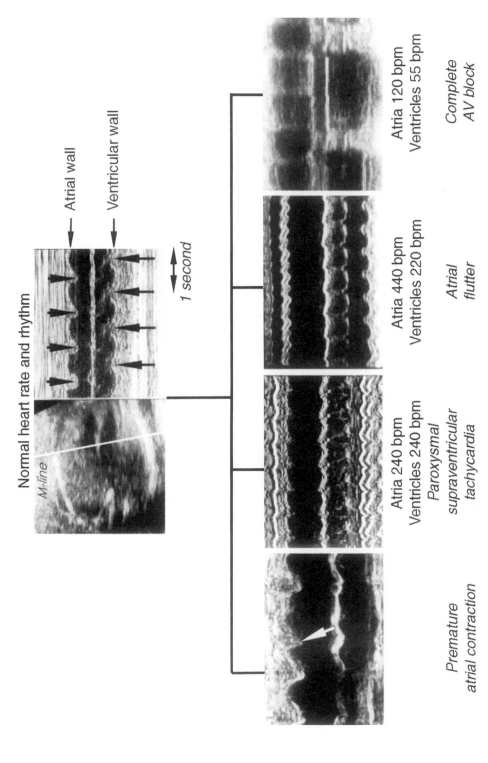

Figure 12 Cardiac dysrhythmias

5

Pulmonary abnormalities

CYSTIC ADENOMATOID MALFORMATION (CAM)

Cystic adenomatoid malformation of the lung is a developmental abnormality arising from an overgrowth of the terminal respiratory bronchioles. The condition may be bilateral involving all lung tissue, but in the majority of cases it is confined to a single lung or lobe. The lesions are either macrocystic (cysts of at least 5 mm in diameter) or microcystic (cysts less than 5 mm in diameter). In 85% of cases, the lesion is unilateral with equal frequency in the right and left lungs and equal frequency in the microcystic and macrocystic types.

Prevalence

Cystic adenomatoid malformation of the lung is found in about 1 in 4000 births.

Etiology

This is a sporadic abnormality. In about 10% of cases, there are other abnormalities, mainly cardiac and renal.

Diagnosis

Prenatal diagnosis is based on the ultrasonographic demonstration of a hyperechogenic pulmonary tumor which is cystic (CAM type 1), mixed (CAM type 2), or solid – microcystic (CAM type 3) (see Figure 13, p. 59). Microcystic disease results in uniform hyperechogenicity of the affected lung tissue. In macrocystic disease, single or multiple cystic spaces may be seen within the thorax. Both microcystic and macrocystic disease may be associated with deviation of the mediastinum; in bilateral disease, the heart may be severely compressed, although not deviated. When there is compression of the heart and major blood vessels in the thorax, fetal hydrops develops. Polyhydramnios is a common feature and this may be a consequence of decreased fetal swallowing of amniotic fluid due to esophageal compression, or increased fluid production by the abnormal lung tissue. Prognostic features for poor outcome include bilateral disease, or unilateral with major lung compression causing pulmonary hypoplasia, and development of hydrops fetalis irrespective of the type of the lesion.

Prognosis

Bilateral disease is lethal either *in utero*, due to progressive hydrops, or in the neonatal period. Isolated unilateral cystic adenomatoid malformation without hydrops is associated with a good prognosis; in about 70% of cases, the relative size of the fetal tumor remains stable, in 20% of cases there is antenatal shrinkage or resolution, and in 10% of cases there is progressive increase in mediastinal compression. In symptomatic neonates, thoracotomy and lobectomy are carried out and survival is about 90%. It is uncertain whether surgery is also needed for asymptomatic neonates.

Fetal therapy

Large intrathoracic cysts causing major mediastinal shift and associated hydrops can be treated effectively by the insertion of thoraco-amniotic shunts. The role of more invasive intervention, such as hysterotomy and excision of solid tumors in cases of fetal hydrops, remains to be defined. Although good results have been reported after such surgery in a small number of cases, the potential risks to the mother both during the pregnancy and in subsequent confinements should not be underestimated.

DIAPHRAGMATIC HERNIA

Development of the diaphragm is usually completed by the 9th week of gestation. In the presence of a defective diaphragm, there is herniation of the abdominal viscera into the thorax at about 10–12 weeks, when the intestines return to the abdominal cavity from the umbilical cord. However, at least in some cases, intrathoracic herniation of viscera may be delayed until the second or third trimester of pregnancy.

Prevalence

Diaphragmatic hernia is found in about 1 per 4000 births.

Etiology

Diaphragmatic hernia is usually a sporadic abnormality. However, in about 50% of affected fetuses there are associated chromosomal abnormalities (mainly trisomy 18, trisomy 13 and Pallister–Killian syndrome – mosaicism for tetrasomy 12p), other defects (mainly craniospinal defects, including spina bifida, hydrocephaly and the otherwise rare iniencephaly, and cardiac abnormalities) and genetic syndromes (such as Fryns syndrome, de Lange syndrome and Marfan syndrome).

Diagnosis

Prenatally, the diaphragm is imaged by ultrasonography as an echo-free space between the thorax and abdomen. Diaphragmatic hernia can be diagnosed by the ultrasonographic demonstration of stomach and intestines (90% of the cases) or liver (50%) in the thorax and the associated mediastinal shift to the opposite side. Herniated abdominal contents, associated with a left-sided diaphragmatic hernia, are easy to demonstrate because the echo-free fluid-filled stomach and small bowel contrast dramatically with the more echogenic fetal lung. In contrast, a right-sided hernia is more difficult to identify because the echogenicity of the fetal liver is similar to that of the lung, and visualization of the gall bladder in the right side of the fetal chest may be the only way of making the diagnosis. Polyhydramnios (usually after 25 weeks) is found in about 75% of cases and this may be the consequence of impaired fetal swallowing due to compression of the esophagus by the herniated abdominal organs. The main differential diagnosis is from cystic lung disease, such as cystic adenomatoid malformation or mediastinal cystic processes, e.g. neuroenteric cysts, bronchogenic cysts and thymic cysts. In these cases, a fluid-filled structure causing mediastinal shift may be present within the chest. However, in contrast to diaphragmatic hernia, the upper abdominal anatomy is normal.

Antenatal prediction of pulmonary hypoplasia remains one of the challenges of prenatal diagnosis because this would be vital in both counselling parents and also in selecting those cases that may benefit from prenatal surgery. Poor prognostic signs are, first, increased nuchal translucency thickness at 10–14 weeks, second, intrathoracic herniation of abdominal viscera before 20 weeks, and, third, severe mediastinal compression suggested by an abnormal ratio in the size of the cardiac ventricles and the development of polyhydramnios.

Prognosis

In the human, the bronchial tree is fully developed by the 16th week of gestation, at which time the full adult number of airways is established. The alveoli continue to develop even after birth, increasing in number and size until the growth of the chest wall is completed in adulthood. The growth of blood vessels supplying the acinus (intra-acinar vessels) parallels alveolar development, while the growth of pre-acinar vessels follows the development of the airways. In diaphragmatic hernia, the reduced thoracic space available to the developing lung leads to reduction in airways, alveoli and arteries. Furthermore, there is an increase in arterial medial wall thickness and extension of muscle peripherally into the small pre-acinar arteries, offering an explanation for the pulmonary hypertension and persistent fetal circulation observed after neonatal repair. Thus, although isolated diaphragmatic hernia is an anatomically simple defect, which is easily correctable, the mortality rate is about 50%. The main cause of death is hypoxemia due to pulmonary hypertension, resulting from the abnormal development of the pulmonary vascular bed.

Fetal therapy

Extensive animal studies have suggested that pulmonary hypoplasia and hypertension due to intrathoracic compression are reversible by *in utero* surgical repair. However, such therapy is likely to have limited success in the human because the bronchial tree is fully developed by the 16th week of gestation. For a fetus with a sonographically demonstrable large diaphragmatic hernia at 16–18 weeks, irreversible maldevelopment of the bronchial tree and vasculature is likely. However, in fetuses with a diaphragmatic defect which allows the intrathoracic herniation of abdominal viscera only after mid-gestation (when the bronchial tree and pre-acinar vessels are fully developed), pre-natal correction, by allowing further development of the alveoli and intra-acinar vessels, may well prevent pulmonary hypoplasia and neonatal death. In a few cases of diaphragmatic hernia, hysterotomy and fetal surgery have been carried out but this intervention has now be abandoned in favor of minimally invasive surgery. Animal studies have demonstrated that obstruction of the trachea results in expansion of the fetal lungs by retained pulmonary secretions. Endoscopic occlusion of the fetal trachea has also been carried out in human fetuses with diaphragmatic hernia, but the number of cases is too small for useful conclusions to be drawn as to the effectiveness of such treatment.

PLEURAL EFFUSIONS

Fetal pleural effusions, which may be unilateral (usually right-sided) or bilateral, may be an isolated finding or they occur in association with generalized edema and ascites (see p. 115).

Prognosis

Irrespective of the underlying cause, infants affected by pleural effusions usually present in the neonatal period with severe, and often fatal, respiratory insufficiency. This is either a direct result of pulmonary compression caused by the effusions, or due to pulmonary hypoplasia secondary to chronic intrathoracic compression. The overall mortality of neonates with pleural effusions is 25%, with a range from 15% in infants with isolated pleural effusions to 95% in those with gross hydrops. The mortality rate in cases of antenatally diagnosed chylothorax is about 50%. Isolated pleural effusions in the fetus may either resolve spontaneously or they can be treated effectively after birth. Nevertheless, in some cases, severe and chronic compression of the fetal lungs can result in pulmonary hypoplasia and neonatal death. In others, mediastinal compression leads to the development of hydrops and polyhydramnios, which are associated with a high risk of premature delivery and perinatal death.

Fetal therapy

Attempts at prenatal therapy by repeated thoracocenteses for drainage of pleural effusions have been generally unsuccessful in reversing the hydropic state, because the fluid reaccumulates within 24–48 h of drainage. A better approach is chronic drainage by the insertion of thoracoamniotic shunts. This is useful both for diagnosis and treatment. First, the diagnosis of an underlying cardiac abnormality or other intrathoracic lesion may become apparent only after effective decompression and return of the mediastinum to its normal position. Second, it can reverse fetal hydrops, resolve polyhydramnios and thereby reduce the risk of preterm delivery, and may prevent pulmonary hypoplasia. Third, it may be useful in the prenatal diagnosis of pulmonary hypoplasia because, in such cases, the lungs often fail to expand after shunting. Furthermore, it may help to distinguish between hydrops due to primary accumulation of pleural effusions, in which case the ascites and skin edema may resolve after shunting, and other causes of hydrops such as infection, in which drainage of the effusions does not prevent worsening of the hydrops. Survival after thoracoamniotic shunting is more than 90% in fetuses with isolated pleural effusions and about 50% in those with hydrops.

SEQUESTRATION OF THE LUNGS

In lung sequestration, a portion of the lung develops without connection to the airways. The blood supply to the abnormal lung tissue is through arteries that arise from the descending aorta rather than from the pulmonary artery. This condition is classically divided in the radiological literature into intralobar (about 75%) and extralobar (about 25%), but the difference (which is based on the presence or absence of a separate pleural covering from the normal lung) cannot be accurately determined with prenatal ultrasound.

Prevalence

Sequestration of the lungs is rare and the prevalence is less than 5% of congenital pulmonary abnormalities.

Etiology

Sequestration of the lungs is a sporadic abnormality.

Diagnosis

The sequestrated portion of the lung appears as a homogeneous, brightly echogenic mass in the lower lobes of the lungs or in the upper abdomen (infradiaphragmatic sequestration). The diagnosis is confirmed by color Doppler demonstration that the vascular supply of the sequestered lobe arises from the abdominal aorta. Large lung sequestration may act as an arteriovenous fistula and cause high-output heart failure and hydrops. Intralobar sequestrations are usually isolated, whereas more than 50% of extralobar sequestrations are associated with other abnormalities (mainly diaphragmatic hernia and cardiac defects).

Prognosis

Postnatal outcome depends on the presence of associated abnormalities, and hemodynamic disturbances. In general, intralobar sequestration has an excellent prognosis, whereas extralobar sequestration has a poor prognosis because of the high incidence of other defects and hydrops.

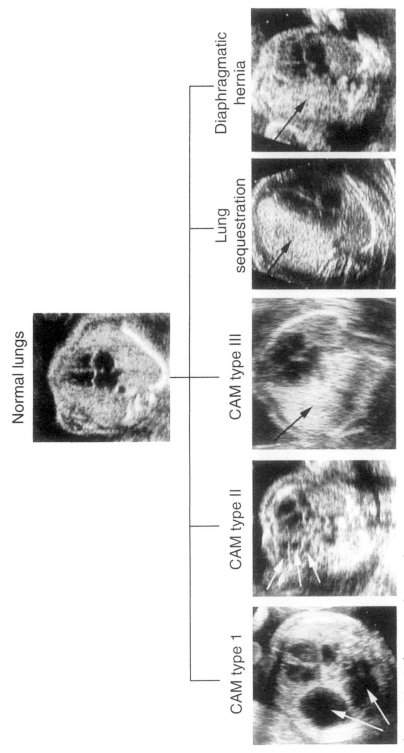

Figure 13 Pulmonary abnormalities

6

Anterior abdominal wall

NORMAL SONOGRAPHIC ANATOMY

Normal development of the anterior abdominal wall depends on the fusion of four ectomesodermic folds (cephalic, caudal and two lateral). At 8–10 weeks of gestation, all fetuses demonstrate herniation of the mid-gut that is visualized as a hyperechogenic mass in the base of the umbilical cord; retraction into the abdominal cavity occurs at 10–12 weeks and is completed by 11 weeks and 5 days. The integrity of the abdominal wall should always be demonstrated; this can be achieved by transverse scans demonstrating the insertion of the umbilical cord. It is also important to visualize the urinary bladder within the fetal pelvis, because this rules out exstrophy of the bladder and of the cloaca.

EXOMPHALOS

Exomphalos results from failure of normal embryonic regression of the mid-gut from the umbilical stalk into the abdominal celom. The abdominal contents, including intestines and liver or spleen covered by a sac of parietal peritoneum and amnion, are herniated into the base of the umbilical cord. Less often there is an associated failure in the cephalic embryonic fold, resulting in the pentalogy of Cantrell (upper mid-line omphalocele, anterior diaphragmatic hernia, sternal cleft, ectopia cordis and intracardiac defects) or failure of the caudal fold, in which case the omphalocele may be associated with exstrophy of the bladder or cloaca, imperforate anus, colonic atresia and sacral vertebral defects. The Beckwith–Wiedemann syndrome (usually sporadic and occasionally familial syndrome with a birth prevalence of about 1 in 14 000) is the association of omphalocele, macrosomia, organomegaly and macroglossia; in some cases there is mental handicap, which is thought to be secondary to inadequately treated hypoglycemia. About 5% of affected individuals develop tumors during childhood, most commonly nephroblastoma and hepatoblastoma.

Prevalence

Exomphalos is found in about 1 per 4000 births.

Etiology

The majority of cases are sporadic and the recurrence risk is usually less than 1%. However, in some cases, there may be an associated genetic syndrome. Chromosomal abnormalities (mainly trisomy 18 or 13) are found in about 50% of cases at 12 weeks, 30% of cases at mid-gestation and in 15% of neonates. Similarly, in Beckwith–Wiedemann syndrome, most cases are sporadic, although autosomal dominant, recessive, X-linked and polygenic patterns of inheritance have been described.

Diagnosis

The diagnosis of exomphalos is based on the demonstration of the mid-line anterior abdominal wall defect, the herniated sac with its visceral contents and the umbilical cord insertion at the apex of the sac (see Figure 14, p. 65). Ultrasonographic examination should be directed towards defining the extent of the lesion and exclusion of other malformations.

Prognosis

Exomphalos is a correctable malformation in which survival depends primarily on whether or not other malformations or chromosomal defects are present. For isolated lesions, the survival rate after surgery is about 90%. The mortality is much higher with cephalic fold defects than with lateral and caudal defects.

GASTROSCHISIS

In gastroschisis, the primary body folds and the umbilical ring develop normally and evisceration of the intestine occurs through a small abdominal wall defect located just lateral and usually to the right of an intact umbilical cord. The loops of intestine lie uncovered in the amniotic fluid and become thickened, edematous and matted.

Prevalence

Gastroschisis is found in about 1 per 4000 births.

Etiology

This is a sporadic abnormality. Associated chromosomal abnormalities are rare, and, although other malformations are found in 10–30% of the cases, these are mainly gut atresias, probably due to gut strangulation and infarction *in utero*.

Diagnosis

Prenatal diagnosis is based on the demonstration of the normally situated umbilicus and the herniated loops of intestine, which are free-floating and widely separated (see Figure 14, p. 65). About 30% of fetuses are growth-restricted but the diagnosis can be difficult because gastroschisis as such is associated with a small abdominal circumference.

Prognosis

Postoperative survival is about 90%; mortality is usually the consequence of short gut syndrome. In this condition, the infants require total parenteral nutrition and they usually die within the first 4 years of life from liver disease.

BODY STALK ANOMALY

This abnormality is characterized by the presence of a major abdominal wall defect, severe kyphoscoliosis and a rudimentary umbilical cord.

Prevalence

Body stalk anomaly is found in about 1 per 10 000 pregnancies.

Etiology

This is a sporadic abnormality. The pathogenesis is uncertain but possible causes include abnormal folding of the trilaminar embryo during the first 4 weeks of development, early amnion rupture with amniotic band syndrome, and early generalized compromise of embryonic blood flow.

Diagnosis

The ultrasonographic features are a major abdominal wall defect, severe kyphoscoliosis and a short umbilical cord. In the first trimester, it is possible to demonstrate that part of the fetal body is in the amniotic cavity and the other part is in the celomic cavity. The findings suggest that early amnion rupture before obliteration of the celomic cavity is a possible cause of the syndrome.

Prognosis

This is a lethal abnormality.

BLADDER EXSTROPHY AND CLOACAL EXSTROPHY

Bladder exstrophy is a defect of the caudal fold of the anterior abdominal wall; a small defect may cause epispadias alone, whilst a large defect leads to exposure of the posterior bladder wall. In cloacal exstrophy, both the urinary and gastrointestinal tracts are involved. Cloacal exstrophy (also referred to as OEIS complex) is the association of an omphalocele, exstrophy of the bladder, imperforated anus, and spinal defects such as meningomyelocele. The hemibladders are on either side of the intestines.

Prevalence

Bladder exstrophy is found in 1 per 30 000 births and cloacal exstrophy is found in about 1 in per 200 000 births.

Etiology

Both bladder exstrophy and cloacal exstrophy are sporadic abnormalities.

Diagnosis

Bladder exstrophy should be suspected when, in the presence of normal amniotic fluid, the fetal bladder is not visualized (the filling cycle of the bladder is normally in the range of 15 min); an echogenic mass is seen protruding from the lower abdominal wall, in close association with the umbilical arteries (see Figure 14, p. 65). In cloacal exstrophy, the findings are similar to bladder exstrophy (large infraumbilical defect that extends to the pelvis), but a posterior anomalous component (meningomyelocele) is present. Other findings include single umbilical artery, ascites, vertebral anomalies, club foot and ambiguous genitalia (in boys, the penis is divided and duplicated).

Prognosis

With aggresive reconstructive bladder, bowel and genital surgery, survival is more than 80%. Although it has been suggested that gender re-assignment to females should occur, psychological follow-ups of such patients suggest that both male and females with this condition are capable of a normal lifestyle with normal intelligence, although some form of urinary tract diversion is required for all. Furthermore, both sexes have been reported to be fertile after surgery.

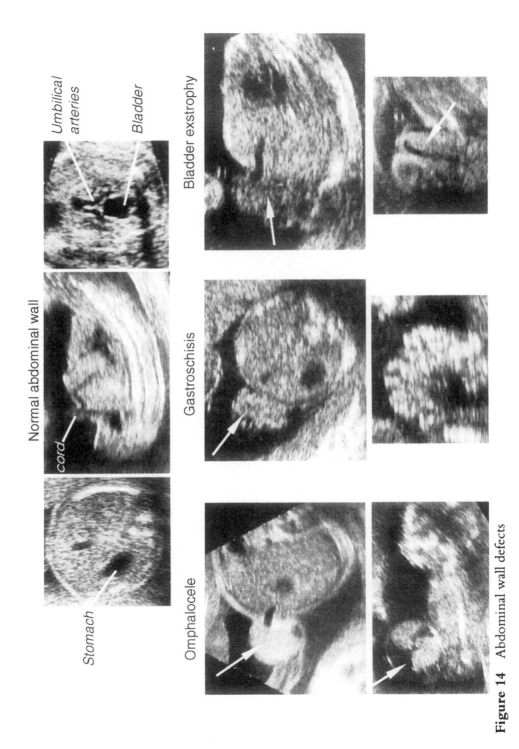

Umbilical arteries

Bladder

Normal abdominal wall

cord

Stomach

Bladder exstrophy

Gastroschisis

Omphalocele

Figure 14 Abdominal wall defects

7

Gastrointestinal tract

NORMAL SONOGRAPHIC ANATOMY

Sonographically, the fetal stomach is visible from 9 weeks of gestation as a sonolucent cystic structure in the upper left quadrant of the abdomen. The bowel is normally uniformly echogenic until the third trimester of pregnancy, when prominent meconium-filled loops of large bowel are commonly seen. The liver comprises most of the upper abdomen and the left lobe is greater in size than the right due to its greater supply of oxygenated blood. The gall bladder is seen as an ovoid cystic structure to the right and below the intrahepatic portion of the umbilical vein. The spleen may also be visualized in a transverse plane posterior and to the left of the fetal stomach. The abdominal circumference should be measured in a cross-section of the abdomen demonstrating the stomach and portal sinus of the liver (see Figure 15, p. 76). The visceral situs should be assessed, by demonstrating the relative position of the stomach, hepatic vessels, abdominal aorta and inferior vena cava.

ESOPHAGEAL ATRESIA

Esophageal atresia and tracheoesophageal fistulae, found in about 90% of cases, result from failure of the primitive foregut to divide into the anterior trachea and posterior esophagus, which normally occurs during the 4th week of gestation.

Prevalence

Esophageal atresia is found in about 1 in 3000 births.

Etiology

Esophageal atresia and tracheoesophageal fistulae are sporadic abnormalities. Chromosomal abnormalities (mainly trisomy 18 or 21) are found in about 20% of fetuses. Other major defects, mainly cardiac, are found in about 50% of the cases. Tracheoesophageal fistulae may be seen as part of the VATER association (vertebral and ventricular septal defects, anal atresia, tracheoesophageal fistula, renal anomalies, radial dysplasia and single umbilical artery).

Diagnosis

Prenatally, the diagnosis of esophageal atresia is suspected when, in the presence of polyhydramnios (usually after 25 weeks), repeated ultrasonographic examinations fail to demonstrate the fetal stomach (see Figure 15, p. 76); however, gastric secretions may be sufficient to distend the stomach and make it visible. If there is an associated fistula, the stomach may look normal. Occasionally (after 25 weeks), the dilated proximal esophageal pouch can be seen as an elongated upper mediastinal and retrocardiac anechoic structure. The differential diagnosis for the combination of absent stomach and polyhydramnios includes intrathoracic compression, by conditions such as diaphragmatic hernia, and muscular–skeletal anomalies causing inability of the fetus to swallow.

Prognosis

Survival is primarily dependent on gestation at delivery and the presence of other anomalies. Thus, for babies with an isolated tracheoesophageal fistula, born after 32 weeks, when an early diagnosis is made, avoiding reflux and aspiration pneumonitis, postoperative survival is more than 95%.

DUODENAL ATRESIA

At 5 weeks of embryonic life, the lumen of the duodenum is obliterated by proliferating epithelium. The patency of the lumen is usually restored by the 11th week and failure of vacuolization may lead to stenosis or atresia. Duodenal obstruction can also be caused by compression from the surrounding annular pancreas or by peritoneal fibrous bands.

Prevalence

Duodenal atresia is found in about 1 per 5000 births.

Etiology

Duodenal atresia is a sporadic abnormality, although, in some cases, there is an autosomal recessive pattern of inheritance. Approximately half of fetuses with duodenal atresia have associated abnormalities, including trisomy 21 (in about 40% of fetuses) and skeletal defects (vertebral and rib anomalies, sacral agenesis, radial abnormalities and talipes), gastrointestinal abnormalities (esophageal atresia/tracheoesophageal fistula, intestinal malrotation, Meckel's diverticulum and anorectal atresia), cardiac and renal defects.

Diagnosis

Prenatal diagnosis is based on the demonstration of the characteristic 'double bubble' appearance of the dilated stomach and proximal duodenum, commonly associated with polyhydramnios (see Figure 15, p. 76). However, obstruction due to an central web may result in only a 'single bubble', representing the fluid-filled stomach. Continuity of the duodenum with the stomach should be demonstrated to differentiate a distended duodenum from other cystic masses, including choledochal or hepatic cysts. Although the characteristic 'double bubble' can be seen as early as 20 weeks, it is usually not diagnosed until after 25 weeks, suggesting that the fetus is unable to swallow a sufficient volume of amniotic fluid for bowel dilatation to occur before the end of the second trimester of pregnancy.

Prognosis

Survival after surgery in cases with isolated duodenal atresia is more than 95%.

INTESTINAL OBSTRUCTION

Intestinal obstructions are either intrinsic or extrinsic. Intrinsic lesions result from absent (atresia) or partial (stenosis) recanalization of the intestine. In cases of atresia, the two segments of the gut may be either completely separated or connected by a fibrous cord. In cases of stenosis, the lumen of the gut is narrowed or the two intestinal segments are separated by a septum with a central diaphragm. Apple-peel atresia is characterized by absence of a vast segment of the small bowel, which can include distal duodenum, the entire jejunum and proximal ileus. Extrinsic obstructions are caused by malrotation of the colon with volvulus, peritoneal bands, meconium ileus, and agangliosis (Hirschsprung's disease). The most frequent site of small bowel obstruction is distal ileus (35%), followed by proximal jejunum (30%), distal jejunum (20%), proximal ileus (15%). In about 5% of cases, obstructions occur in multiple sites. Anorectal atresia results from abnormal division of the cloaca during the 9th week of development.

Prevalence

Intestinal obstruction is found in about 1 per 2000 births; in about half of the cases, there is small bowel obstruction and in the other half anorectal atresia.

Etiology

Although the condition is usually sporadic, in multiple intestinal atresia, familial cases have been described. Associated abnormalities and chromosomal defects are rare. In contrast with anorectal atresia, associated defects such as genitourinary, vertebral, cardiovascular and gastrointestinal anomalies are found in about 80% of cases.

Diagnosis

The lumens of the small bowel and colon do not normally exceed 7 mm and 20 mm, respectively. Diagnosis of obstruction is usually made quite late in pregnancy (after 25 weeks), as dilatation of the intestinal lumen is slow and progressive. Jejunal and ileal obstructions are imaged as multiple fluid-filled loops of bowel in the abdomen (see Figure 15, p. 76). The abdomen is usually distended and active peristalsis may be observed. If bowel perforation occurs, transient ascites, meconium peritonitis and meconium pseudocysts may ensue. Polyhydramnios (usually after 25 weeks) is common, especially with proximal obstructions. Similar bowel appearances and polyhydramnios may be found in fetuses with Hirschsprung's disease, the megacystis–microcolon–intestinal hypoperistalsis syndrome and congenital chloride diarrhea. When considering a diagnosis of small bowel obstruction, care should be taken to exclude renal tract abnormalities and other intra-abdominal cysts such as mesenteric, ovarian or duplication cysts. In anorectal atresia, prenatal diagnosis is usually difficult because the proximal bowel may not demonstrate significant dilatation and the amniotic fluid volume is usually normal; occasionally calcified intraluminal meconium in the fetal pelvis may be seen.

Prognosis

Infants with bowel obstruction typically present in the early neonatal period with symptoms of vomiting and abdominal distention. The prognosis is related to the gestational age at delivery, the presence of associated abnormalities and site of obstruction. In those born after 32 weeks with isolated obstruction requiring resection of only a short segment of bowel, survival is more than 95%. Loss of large segments of bowel can lead to short gut syndrome, which is a lethal condition.

HIRSCHSPRUNG'S DISEASE

Hirschsprung's disease is characterized by congenital absence of intramural parasympathetic nerve ganglia in a segment of the colon. It derives from failure of migration of neuroblasts from the neural crest to the bowel segments, which generally occurs between the 6th and 12th weeks of gestation. Another theory suggests that the disease is caused by degeneration of normally migrated neuroblasts during either pre- or postnatal life.

Prevalence

The disease occurs in about 1 in 3000 births.

Etiology

It is considered to be a sporadic disease, although in about 5% of cases there is a familial inheritance. In a small number of cases, Hirschsprung's disease is associated with trisomy 21.

Diagnosis

The aganglionic segment is unable to transmit a peristaltic wave, and therefore meconium accumulates and causes dilatation of the lumen of the bowel. The ultrasound appearance is similar to that of anorectal atresia, when the affected segment is colon or rectum. Polyhydramnios and dilatation of the loops are present in the case of small bowel involvement; on this occasion, it is not different from other types of obstruction.

Prognosis

Postnatal surgery is aimed at removing the affected segment and this may be a two-stage procedure with temporary colostomy. Neonatal mortality is approximately 20%.

MECONIUM PERITONITIS

Intrauterine perforation of the bowel may lead to a local sterile chemical peritonitis, with the development of a dense calcified mass of fibrous tissue sealing off the perforation. Bowel perforation usually occurs proximal to some form of obstruction, although this cannot always be demonstrated.

Etiology

Intestinal stenosis or atresia and meconium ileus account for 65% of the cases. Other causes include volvulus and Meckel's diverticulum. Meconium ileus is the impaction of abnormally thick and sticky meconium in the distal ileum, and, in the majority of cases, this is due to cystic fibrosis.

Prevalence

Meconium peritonitis is found in about 1 in 3000 births.

Diagnosis

The diagnosis should be considered if the fetal bowel is observed to be dilated or whenever an area of fetal intra-abdominal hyperechogenicity is detected. The likelihood of perforation is increased if a thin rim of ascites is also demonstrated. The differential diagnosis of hyperechogenic bowel includes:

(1) Intra-amniotic hemorrhage;

(2) Early ascites;

(3) Fetal hypoxia;

(4) Meconium peritonitis; and

(5) Cystic fibrosis.

Meconium ileus and hyperechogenic fetal bowel at 16–18 weeks of gestation may be present in 75% of fetuses with cystic fibrosis. The prevalence of cystic fibrosis in fetuses with prenatal diagnosis of intestinal obstruction may be about 10%. Therefore, when other causes of bowel hyperechogenicity have been excluded, DNA studies for cystic fibrosis should be considered.

Prognosis

Meconium peritonitis is associated with a more than 50% mortality in the neonatal period.

HEPATOSPLENOMEGALY

The fetal liver and spleen can be measured by ultrasonography. Causes of hepatosplenomegaly include immune and non-immune hydrops, congenital infection and metabolic disorders, and it is seen in Beckwith–Wiedemann and Zellweger syndromes. Hepatic enlargement may also be caused by hemangioma, which is usually hypoechogenic, or hepatoblastoma (the most frequent malignant tumor in fetal life), in which there are areas of calcification.

HEPATIC CALCIFICATIONS

Hepatic calcifications are echogenic foci in the parenchyma or the capsule of the liver.

Prevalence

Hepatic calcifications are found at mid-trimester ultrasonography in about 1 per 2000 fetuses.

Etiology

The vast majority of cases are idiopathic but, in a few cases, hepatic calcifications have been found in association with congenital infections and chromosomal abnormalities.

Diagnosis

Solitary or multiple echogenic foci (1–2 mm in diameter) are observed within the substance of the liver or in the capsule.

Prognosis

This depends on the presence of associated infection or chromosomal defects. Isolated foci are of no pathological significance.

ABDOMINAL CYSTS

Abdominal cystic masses are frequent findings at ultrasound examination. Renal tract anomalies or dilated bowel are the most common explanations, although cystic structures may arise from the biliary tree, ovaries, mesentery or uterus. The correct diagnosis of these abnormalities may not be possible by ultrasound examination, but the most likely diagnosis is usually suggested by the position of the cyst, its relationship with other structures and the normality of other organs.

Choledochal cysts

Choledochal cysts represent cystic dilatation of the common biliary duct. They are uncommon and their etiology is unknown. Prenatally, the diagnosis may be made ultrasonographically by the demonstration of a cyst in the upper right side of the fetal abdomen. The differential diagnosis includes enteric duplication cyst, liver cysts, situs inversus or duodenal atresia. The absence of polyhydramnios or peristalsis may help to differentiate the condition from bowel disorders. Postnatally, early diagnosis and removal of the cyst may avoid the development of biliary cirrhosis, portal hypertension, calculi formation or adenocarcinoma. The operative mortality is about 10%.

Ovarian cysts

Ovarian cysts are common and they may be found in up to one-third of newborns at autopsy, although they are usually small and asymptomatic. Fetal ovarian cysts are hormone-sensitive (human chorionic gonadotropin from the placenta) and tend to occur after 25 weeks of gestation; they more common in diabetic or rhesus iso-immunized mothers as a result of placental hyperplasia. The majority of cysts are benign and resolve spontaneously in the neonatal period. Potential complications include development of ascites, torsion, infarction or rupture. Prenatally, the cysts are usually unilateral and unilocular, although, if the cyst undergoes torsion or hemorrhage, the appearance is complex or solid. Large ovarian cysts can be found in association with polyhydramnios, possibly as a consequence of compression of the bowel. Obstetric management should not be changed, unless an enormous or rapidly enlarging cyst is detected or there is associated polyhydramnios; in these cases, prenatal aspiration may be considered. A difficult differential diagnosis is from hydrometrocolpos, which also presents as a cystic or solid mass arising from the pelvis of a female fetus. Other genitourinary or gastrointestinal anomalies are common and include renal agenesis, polycystic kidneys, esophageal atresia, duodenal atresia and imperforate anus. Most cases are sporadic, although a few cases are genetic, such as the autosomal recessive McKusick–Kaufman syndrome with hydrometrocolpos, polydactyly and congenital heart disease.

Mesenteric or omental cysts

Mesenteric or omental cysts may represent obstructed lymphatic drainage or lymphatic hamartomas. The fluid contents may be serous, chylous or hemorrhagic. Antenatally, the diagnosis is suggested by the finding of a multiseptate or unilocular, usually mid-line, cystic lesion of variable size; a solid appearance may be secondary to hemorrhage. Antenatal aspiration may be considered in cases of massive cysts resulting in thoracic compression. Postnatal management is conservative and surgery is reserved for cases with symptoms of bowel obstruction or acute abdominal pain following torsion or hemorrhage into a cyst. Complete excision of cysts may not be possible because of the proximity of major blood vessels and in up to 20% of cases there is recurrence after surgery. Although malignant change in mesenteric cysts has been described, this is rare.

Hepatic cysts

Hepatic cysts are typically located in the right lobe of the liver. They are quite rare and result from obstruction of the hepatic biliary system. They appear as unilocular, intrahepatic cysts, and they are usually asymptomatic, although rarely may show complications such as infections or hemorrhages. In 30% of the cases of polycystic kidneys (adult type), asymptomatic hepatic cysts may be associated.

Intestinal duplication cysts

These are quite rare, and may be located along the entire gastrointestinal tract. They sonographically appear as tubular or cystic structures of variable size. They may be isolated or associated with other gastrointestinal malformations. Differential diagnosis includes other intra-abdominal cystic structures and also bronchogenic cysts, adenomatoid cystic malformation of the lung and pulmonary sequestration. Thickness of the muscular wall of the cysts and presence of peristalsis may facilitate the diagnosis. Postnatally, surgical removal is carried out.

Anomalies of the umbilical vein

Abnormalities of the umbilical vein, which are very rare, can be divided in three groups:

(1) Persistence of the right umbilical vein with ductus venosus and presence or absence of left umbical vein;

(2) Absence of the ductus venosus with extrahepatic insertion of the umbilical vein; and

(3) Dilated umbilical vein with normal insertion.

Normally, the umbilical vein enters the abdomen almost centrally at the level of the liver and courses on the left of the gallbladder. Persistence of the right umbilical vein is demonstrated by the fact that it is localized on the right of the gallbladder, bending towards the stomach. Color Doppler may help to diagnose these anomalies and may allow the differential diagnosis with other cystic abdominal lesions. Associated anomalies are frequent in anomalies of the first two groups and this influences the prognosis. These anomalies include cardiac, skeletal, gastrointestinal and urinary anomalies. The anomalies of the third group are rarely associated with other anomalies, and prognosis depends on the time at diagnosis and dimension of the varicosity.

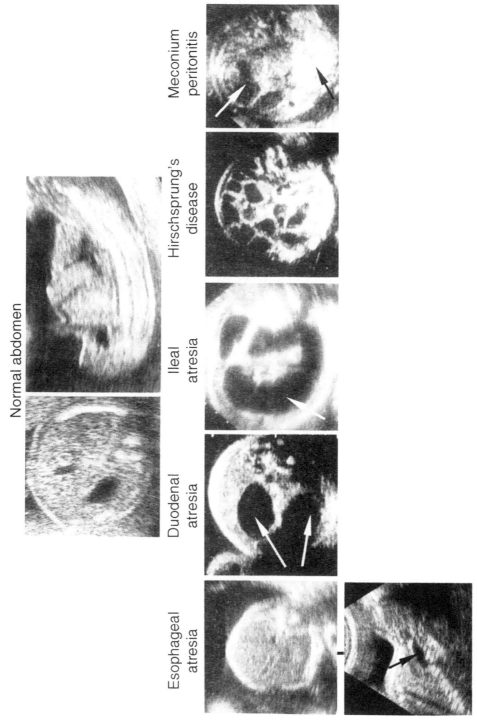

Figure 15 Defects of the gastrointestinal tract

8

Kidneys and urinary tract

NORMAL SONOGRAPHIC ANATOMY

The kidneys and adrenals, located below the level of the stomach, on either side and anterior to the spine, are visible by ultrasonography from as early as 9 weeks of gestation and in all cases from 12 weeks. The renal echogenicity is high at 9 weeks but decreases with gestation; the adrenals appear as translucent structures with an echodense cortex.

Longitudinal and transverse sections of the abdomen can be used to study the kidneys. In a longitudinal scan, kidneys appear as elliptical areas, while on transverse scan they appear as roundish structures at both sides of the spine. The kidneys appear slightly hypoechoic, compared to the liver and bowel loops. At 20 weeks, the kidneys show a hyperechoic capsule and the cortical area is slightly more echogenic than the medulla. With progressing gestation, fat tissue accumulates around the kidneys, enhancing the borders of the kidneys in contrast with the other splanchnic organs. At 26–28 weeks, renal pyramids can be detected, and the arcuate arteries can be seen pulsating in their proximity. Both the renal length and circumference increase with gestation, but the ratio of renal to abdominal circumference remains approximately 30% throughout pregnancy. The anteroposterior diameter of the renal pelvis should be < 5 mm at 15–19 weeks, < 6 mm at 20–29 weeks and < 8 mm at 30–40 weeks. The normal ureters are rarely seen in the absence of distal obstruction or reflux. The fetal bladder can be visualized from the first trimester (in about 80% of fetuses at 11 weeks and more than 90% by 13 weeks); changes in volume over time help to differentiate it from other cystic pelvic structures.

RENAL AGENESIS

Renal agenesis is the consequence of failure of differentiation of the metanephric blastema during the 25–28th day of development and both ureters and kidneys and renal arteries are absent.

Prevalence

Bilateral renal agenesis is found in 1 per 5000 births, while unilateral disease is found in 1 per 2000 births.

Etiology

Renal agenesis is usually an isolated sporadic abnormality but, in a few cases, it may be secondary to a chromosomal abnormality or part of a genetic syndrome (such as Fraser syndrome), or a developmental defect (such as VACTERL association). In non-syndromic cases, the risk of recurrence is approximately 3%. However, in about 15% of cases, one of the parents has unilateral renal agenesis and in these families the risk of recurrence is increased.

Diagnosis

Antenatally, the condition is suspected by the combination of anhydramnios (from 17 weeks) and empty fetal bladder (from as early as 14 weeks). Examination of the renal areas is often hampered by the oligohydramnios and the 'crumpled' position adopted by these fetuses, and care should be taken to avoid the mistaken diagnosis of perirenal fat and large fetal adrenals for the absent kidneys. The differential diagnosis is from preterm rupture of membranes, severe uteroplacental insufficiency and obstructive uropathy or bilateral multicystic or polycystic kidneys. Vaginal sonography with high-frequency, high-resolution probes is useful in these cases. Failure to visualize the renal arteries with color Doppler is another important clue to the diagnosis in dubious cases, both with bilateral and unilateral agenesis. Prenatal diagnosis of unilateral renal agenesis is difficult because there are no major features, such as anhydramnios and empty bladder, to alert the ultrasonographer to the fact that one of the kidneys is absent.

Prognosis

Bilateral renal agenesis is a lethal condition, usually in the neonatal period due to pulmonary hypoplasia. The prognosis with unilateral agenesis is normal.

INFANTILE POLYCYSTIC KIDNEY DISEASE (POTTER TYPE I)

In this condition, the markedly enlarged kidneys are filled with numerous cortical cysts and dilated collecting ducts. The disease has a wide spectrum of renal and hepatic involvement and it is subdivided into perinatal (this is the most common), neonatal, infantile and juvenile types on the basis of the age of onset of the clinical presentation and the degree of renal tubular involvement. Although recurrences tend to be group-specific, we have seen one family in which the four subdivisions were each represented in the four affected infants.

Prevalence

Infantile polycystic kidney disease is found in about 1 per 30 000 births.

Etiology

This is an autosomal recessive condition. The responsible gene is in the short arm of chromosome 6 and prenatal diagnosis in families at risk can be carried out by first-trimester chorion villous sampling.

Diagnosis

Prenatal diagnosis is confined to the types with earlier onset (perinatal and probably the neonatal types) and is based on the demonstration of bilaterally enlarged and homogeneously hyperechogenic kidneys (see Figure 16, p. 85). There is often associated oligohydramnios, but this is not invariably so. These sonographic appearances, however, may not become apparent before 24 weeks of gestation and, therefore, serial scans should be performed for exclusion of the diagnosis.

Prognosis

The perinatal type is lethal either *in utero* or in the neonatal period due to pulmonary hypoplasia. The neonatal type results in death due to renal failure within the 1st year of life. The infantile and juvenile types result in chronic renal failure, hepatic fibrosis and portal hypertension; many cases survive into their teens and require renal transplantation.

MULTICYSTIC DYSPLASTIC KIDNEY DISEASE (POTTER TYPE II)

Multicystic dysplastic kidney disease is thought to be a consequence of either developmental failure of the mesonephric blastema to form nephrons or early obstruction due to urethral or ureteric atresia. The collecting tubules become cystic and the diameter of the cysts determines the size of the kidneys, which may be enlarged or small. Exploration of the renal fossa in some cases reveals no renal artery, renal vein, ureter or cysts, suggesting that renal agenesis and dysplastic kidneys may be at different ends of a spectrum of renal malformation. This is further supported by the finding that, in about 15% of cases with multicystic kidneys, there is contralateral renal agenesis.

Prevalence

Multicystic dysplastic kidney disease is found in about 1 per 1000 births.

Etiology

In the majority of cases, this is a sporadic abnormality but chromosomal abnormalities (mainly trisomy 18), genetic syndromes and other defects (mainly cardiac) are present in about 50% of the cases.

Diagnosis

Ultrasonographically, the kidneys are replaced by multiple irregular cysts of variable size with intervening hyperechogenic stroma (see Figure 16, p. 85). The disorder can be bilateral, unilateral or segmental; if bilateral, there is associated anhydramnios and the bladder is 'absent'.

Prognosis

Bilateral multicystic dysplastic kidney disease is fatal before or soon after birth, due to pulmonary hypoplasia. Unilateral disease is associated with a normal prognosis. There is still controversy in the postnatal management of patients with a multicystic kidney; some urologists advocate prophylactic nephrectomy, but the majority adopt an expectant approach because the kidney gradually shrinks and may disappear. The parents and family should also be scanned to exclude autosomal dominant branchio-to-renal syndrome.

POTTER TYPE III RENAL DYSPLASIA

Potter type III renal dysplasia is characterized by markedly enlarged irregular kidneys with innumerable cysts of variable sizes interspersed among normal or compressed renal parenchyma. It is the common morphological expression of autosomal dominant adult polycystic kidney disease (APKD) and of other Mendelian disorders such as tuberous sclerosis, Jeune syndrome, Sturge–Weber syndrome, Zellweger syndrome, Lawrence Moon Biedl syndrome and Meckel–Gruber syndrome. Both kidneys are generally equally enlarged and only rarely is one involved so slightly that it remains of normal size. One-third of the cases have cysts in the liver, pancreas, spleen or lungs and one-fifth are found to have cerebral aneurysms.

Adult polycystic kidney disease (APKD)

One in 1000 people carry the APKD mutant gene. Adult polycystic kidney disease is usually asymptomatic until the third or fourth decade of life, and, although histological evidence of the disease is likely to be present from intrauterine life, the age of onset of gross morphological changes that are potentially detectable by ultrasonography is uncertain. Rarely, however, kidneys that are anatomically similar may cause death in infancy or early childhood and the condition has been designated as 'adult variety occurring in infancy'.

Prenatal diagnosis by ultrasonography is confined to a few case reports and the kidneys have been described as enlarged and hyperechogenic with or without multiple cysts (see Figure 16, p. 85). Unlike infantile polycystic kidneys, where there is a loss of the corticomedullary junction, in APKD there is accentuation of this junction. The amniotic fluid volume is either normal or reduced. The kidney size is usually smaller than that of the infant polycystic kidneys. In counselling affected parents with APKD, it should be emphasized that the prenatal demonstration of sonographically normal kidneys does not necessarily exclude the possibility of developing polycystic kidneys in adult life. Nevertheless, prenatal diagnosis can now be made from chorion villous sampling and DNA analysis.

OBSTRUCTIVE UROPATHIES

The term 'obstructive uropathy' encompasses a wide variety of different pathological conditions characterized by dilatation of part or all of the urinary tract. When the obstruction is complete and occurs early in fetal life, renal hypoplasia (deficiency in total nephron population) and dysplasia (Potter type II; formation of abnormal nephrons and mesenchymal stroma) ensue. On the other hand, where intermittent obstruction allows for normal renal development, or when it occurs in the second half of pregnancy, hydronephrosis will result and the severity of the renal damage will depend on the degree and duration of the obstruction. Dilatation of the fetal urinary tract frequently, but not absolutely, signifies obstruction. Conversely, a fetus with obstruction may not have any urinary tract dilatation.

Hydronephrosis

Varying degrees of pelvicalyceal dilatation are found in about 1% of fetuses. Mild hydronephrosis or pyelectasia is defined by the presence of an anteroposterior diameter of the pelvis of > 4 mm at 15–19 weeks, > 5 mm at 20–29 weeks and > 7 mm at 30–40 weeks. Transient hydronephrosis may be due to relaxation of smooth muscle of the urinary tract by the high levels of circulating maternal hormones, or maternal–fetal overhydration. In the majority of cases, the condition remains stable or resolves in the neonatal period. In about 20% of cases, there may be an underlying ureteropelvic junction obstruction or vesicoureteric reflux that requires postnatal follow-up and possible surgery.

Moderate hydronephrosis, characterized by an anteroposterior pelvic diameter of more than 10 mm and pelvicalyceal dilatation, is usually progressive and in more than 50% of cases surgery is necessary during the first 2 years of life.

Ureteropelvic junction obstruction

This is usually sporadic and, although in some cases there is an anatomic cause, such as ureteral valves, in most instances the underlying cause is thought to be functional. In 80% of cases, the condition is unilateral. Prenatal diagnosis is based on the demonstration of hydronephrosis in the absence of dilated ureters and bladder. The degree of pelvicalyceal dilatation is variable and, occasionally, perinephric urinomas and urinary ascites may be present. Postnatally, renal function is assessed by serial isotope imaging studies and, if there is deterioration, pyeloplasty is performed. However, the majority of infants have moderate or good function and can be managed expectantly.

Ureterovesical junction obstruction

This is a sporadic abnormality characterized by hydronephrosis and hydroureter in the presence of a normal bladder. The dilated ureter is tortuous, and on ultrasound appears as a collection of cysts of variable size, localized between the renal pelvis, which is variably dilated, and the bladder, which is of normal morphology and dimensions. The etiology is diverse, including ureteric stricture or atresia, retrocaval ureter, vascular obstruction, valves, diverticulum, ureterocele, and vesicoureteral reflux. Ureteroceles (visible as a thin-walled and fluid-filled small circular area inside the bladder) are usually found in association with duplication of the collecting system. In ureteral duplication, the upper pole moiety characteristically obstructs and the lower one refluxes. The dilated upper pole may enlarge to displace the non-dilated lower pole inferiorly and laterally.

Vesicoureteric reflux

This sporadic abnormality is suspected when intermittent dilatation of the upper urinary tract over a short period of time is seen on ultrasound scanning. Occasionally, in massive vesicoureteric reflux without obstruction, the bladder appears persistently dilated because it empties but rapidly refills with refluxed urine. Primary megaureter can be distinguished from ureterovesical junction obstruction by the absence of significant hydronephrosis.

Megacystis–microcolon–intestinal hypoperistalsis syndrome (MMIHS)

This is a sporadic abnormality characterized by a massively dilated bladder and hydronephrosis in the presence of normal or increased amniotic fluid; the fetuses are usually female. There is associated shortening and dilatation of the proximal small bowel, and microcolon with absent or ineffective peristalsis. The condition is usually lethal due to bowel and renal dysfunction.

Urethral obstruction

Urethral obstruction can be caused by urethral agenesis, persistence of the cloaca, urethral stricture or posterior urethral valves. Posterior urethral valves occur only in males and are the commonest cause of bladder outlet obstruction. The condition is sporadic and is found in about 1 in 3000 male fetuses. With posterior urethral valves, there is usually incomplete or intermittent obstruction of the urethra, resulting in an enlarged and hypertrophied bladder with varying degrees of hydroureters, hydronephrosis, a spectrum of renal hypoplasia and dysplasia, oligohydramnios and pulmonary hypoplasia. In some cases, there is associated urinary ascites from rupture of the bladder or transudation of urine into the peritoneal cavity.

Fetal therapy for obstructive uropathy

In fetal lamb, ureteric ligation during the first half of gestation results in dysplastic kidneys, whereas, in the second half of pregnancy, ureteric ligation is associated with the development of hydronephrosis but preservation of renal architecture. Ligation of the urethra and urachus in fetal lambs at 100 days of gestation causes severe hydronephrosis and pulmonary hypoplasia; decompression by suprapubic cystostomy at 120 days' gestation reduces the urinary tract dilatation and improves the survival rate. Similarly, ureteric ligation at 65 days of gestation produces renal dysplasia, and subsequent decompression prior to term prevents renal dysplasia and produces reversible post-obstructive changes; the degree of renal damage is proportional to the length of time for which the obstruction existed.

Encouraged by the results of these animal studies, and on the assumption that unrelieved obstruction causes progressive renal and pulmonary damage, several investigators in the 1980s performed *in utero* decompression of the urinary tract in the human, either by open surgical diversion or by the ultrasound-guided insertion of suprapubic vesico-amniotic catheters. Although these techniques demonstrated the feasibility of intrauterine surgery, they did not provide conclusive evidence that such intervention improves renal or pulmonary function beyond what can be achieved by postnatal surgery. It is possible that, in a few selected cases, intrauterine intervention may be beneficial.

Assessment of fetal renal function

Antenatal evaluation of renal function relies on a combination of ultrasonographic findings and analysis of fetal urine obtained by urodochocentesis or pyelocentesis. Poor prognostic signs are:

(1) The presence of bilateral multicystic or severely hydronephrotic kidneys with echogenic kidneys, suggestive of renal dysplasia;

(2) Anhydramnios implying complete urethral obstruction; and

(3) High urinary sodium, calcium and β2 microglobulin levels.

Potential candidates for intrauterine surgery are fetuses with bilateral moderately severe pelvicalyceal dilatation and normal cortical echogenicity, or severe megacystis and oligohydramnios, or normal levels of urinary sodium, calcium and β2 microglobulin.

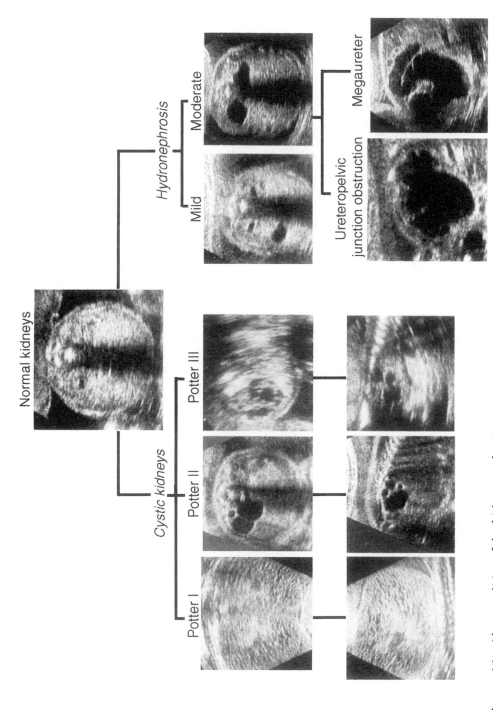

Figure 16   Abnormalities of the kidneys and urinary tract

9

Skeleton

Gianluigi Pilu and Roberto Romero

NORMAL SONOGRAPHIC ANATOMY

Limb buds are first seen by ultrasound at about the 8th week of gestation; the femur and humerus are seen from 9 weeks, the tibia/fibula and radius/ulna from 10 weeks and the digits of the hands and the feet from 11 weeks. All long bones are consistently seen from 11 weeks. Body movements (wiggling) are seen at 9 weeks and, by 11 weeks, limbs move about readily. The lengths of the humerus, radius/ulna, femur and tibia/fibula are similar and increase linearly with gestation. At the 18–23-week scan, the three segments of each extremity should be visualized, but it is only necessary to measure the length of one femur. The relationship of leg and foot should also be assessed to rule out clubfoot.

SKELETAL ANOMALIES

Prevalence

Skeletal dysplasia is found in about 1 per 4000 births; about 25% of affected fetuses are stillborn and about 30% die in the neonatal period. The birth prevalences of the most common dysplasias are shown in the Table on the next page.

Classification

The existing nomenclature for skeletal dysplasias is complicated. Some disorders are referred to by eponyms (such as Ellis–Van Creveld syndrome), by Greek terms describing a salient feature of the disease (diastrophic or twisted, metatrophic or changeable) or by a term related to the presumed pathogenesis of the disease (such as osteogenesis imperfecta). The fundamental problem with any classification of skeletal dysplasias is that the pathogenesis of these diseases is largely unknown and, therefore, the current system relies on purely descriptive findings of either clinical or radiological nature. According to the International Nomenclature for Skeletal Dysplasias, the diseases are subdivided into three different groups:

	Birth prevalence
Lethal dysplasias	
Thanatophoric dysplasia	1 in 10 000
Achondrogenesis	1 in 40 000
Osteogenesis imperfecta, type II	1 in 60 000
Congenital hypophosphatasia	1 in 100 000
Chondrodysplasia punctata	1 in 110 000
Non-lethal dysplasias	
Heterozygous achondroplasia	1 in 30 000
Osteogenesis imperfecta, type I	1 in 30 000
Asphyxiating thoracic dysplasia	1 in 70 000

(1) Osteochondrodysplasias (abnormalities of cartilage and / or bone growth and development);

(2) Disorganized development of cartilaginous and fibrous components of the skeleton; and

(3) Idiopathic osteolyses.

Approach to prenatal diagnosis

There is a wide range of rare skeletal dyplasias, each with a specific recurrence risk, dysmorphic expression, and implications for neonatal survival and quality of life. Our knowledge of the *in utero* expression of these syndromes is based on a few case reports and, therefore, in attempting to perform prenatal diagnosis of individual conditions in at-risk families, extrapolation of findings from the perinatal period is often necessary. The incidental discovery of a skeletal dysplasia on routine ultrasound screening, in a pregnancy not known to be at risk of a specific syndrome, necessitates a systematic examination to arrive at the correct diagnosis. All limbs must be evaluated (see Figure 17, p. 97) as to their length, shape, mineralization and movement, and associated abnormalities in other systems, particularly the head, thorax and spine, should be sought.

Assessment of long bones

Shortening of the extremities can involve the entire limb (micromelia, such as achondrogenesis, short-rib polydactyly syndrome, diastrophic dysplasia osteogenesis imperfecta type II), the proximal segment (rhizomelia, such as achondroplasia), the intermediate segment (mesomelia, such as mesomelic dysplasia) or the distal segment (acromelia, such as Ellis–Van Creveld syndrome). The diagnosis of rhizomelia or mesomelia requires comparison of the dimensions of the bones of the leg and forearm with those of the thigh and arm. The femur, however, is abnormally short even in mesomelic dwarfism and, therefore, in our routine fetal abnormality screening, we tend to confine limb measurements to that of the femur. When dealing with pregnancies at risk for a skeletal dysplasia, both segments of all limbs are measured.

The severe limb reductions associated with osteogenesis imperfecta type II, achondrogenesis and thanatophoric, diastrophic, and chondroectodermal dysplasias can be detected by a single measurement of the femur length at 16–18 weeks of gestation. In the case of achondroplasia, however, the diagnosis may not become obvious until 22–24 weeks and, therefore, serial measurements are necessary; homozygous achondroplasia, which is usually lethal, manifests in abnormally short limbs earlier than the heterozygous form.

A minor degree of lateral curvature of the femur is commonly seen in normal fetuses. Pronounced bowing, however, is observed in association with campomelic dysplasia, thanatophoric dwarfism, autosomal dominant osteogenesis imperfecta, achondrogenesis and hypophosphatasia. In the latter, fractures and callus formation may also be detected. Reduced echogenicity of bones, suggestive of hypomineralization, is seen in such disorders as hypophosphatasia, osteogenesis imperfecta and achondrogenesis. The virtual absence of ossification of the spine, characteristic of achondrogenesis, may lead to the erroneous diagnosis of complete spinal agenesis. Similarly, the pronounced clarity with which the cerebral ventricles are imaged, as a result of the poorly mineralized globular cranium in cases of hypophosphatasia, may result in the misdiagnosis of hydrocephalus. Care must be exercised, however, because lesser degrees of hypomineralization may not be detectable.

Isolated limb reduction deformities, such as amelia (complete absence of extremities), acheiria (absence of the hand), phocomelia (seal limb) or aplasia–hypoplasia of the radius or ulna, are often inherited as part of a genetic syndrome (Holt–Oram syndrome, Fanconi pancytopenia, thrombocytopenia with absent radii syndrome) and are readily diagnosible by ultrasonography in an at-risk fetus. Other causes of focal limb loss include the amniotic band syndrome, thalidomide exposure and caudal regression syndrome.

Evaluation of hands and feet

Fetal fingers and toes can be seen, and, with meticulous examination, abnormalities of numbers, shape, movement and attitudes can be recognized. Several skeletal dysplasias feature alterations of the hands and feet. Polydactyly refers to the presence of more than five digits. It is classified as postaxial if the extra digits are on the ulnar or fibular side and preaxial if they are located on the radial or tibial side. Syndactyly refers to soft tissue or bony fusion of adjacent digits. Clinodactyly consists of deviation of a finger(s). Disproportion between hands and feet and the other parts of the extremity may also be a sign of a skeletal dysplasia.

Examination of fetal movements

Maternal perception of fetal movements is usually decreased in fetuses with skeletal dysplasias, such as achondrogenesis and thanatophoric dysplasia. Ultrasonography can aid in the diagnosis of conditions characterized by limitation of flexion or extension of the limbs, such as arthrogryposis and multiple pterygium syndrome.

Evaluation of thoracic dimensions

Several skeletal dysplasias are associated with a small thorax, and chest restriction leads to pulmonary hypoplasia, which is the common cause of death in these conditions (see Figure 18, p. 98). The appropriateness of thoracic dimensions can be assessed by measuring the thoracic circumference at the level of the four-chamber view of the heart and examining the thoracic-to-abdominal circumference ratio, the thoracic-to-head circumference ratio, or the thoracic-to-cardiac circumference ratio.

Skeletal dysplasias associated with a long narrow thorax include asphyxiating thoracic dysplasia (Jeune), chondroectodermal dysplasia (Ellis–Van Creveld), campomelic dysplasia, Jarcho–Levin syndrome, achondrogenesis and hypophosphatasia. Dysplasias with a short thorax include osteogenesis imperfecta (type II), Kniest's dysplasia (metatrophic dysplasia type II) and Pena–Shokeir syndrome. Hypoplastic thorax is found in short-rib polydactyly syndrome (type I, type II), thanatophoric dysplasia, cerebrocostomandibular syndrome, cleidocranial dysostosis syndrome, homozygous achondroplasia, Melnick–Needles syndrome (osteodysplasty), fibrochondrogenesis and otopalatodigital syndrome type II.

Evaluation of the fetal head

Several skeletal dysplasias are associated with defects of membranous ossification and, therefore, affect skull bones. The face should also be examined for the diagnosis of hypertelorism, micrognathia, short upper lip, and abnormalities of the ears.

Diagnostic tests complementary to sonography

Prenatal or postnatal evaluation includes chromosomal studies, biochemical investigations (e.g. hypophosphatasia) and DNA analysis for an increasing number of the osteochondrodysplasias. Postnatally, examination of skeletal radiographs is of particular importance, since the classification of skeletal dysplasias is largely based upon radiographic findings.

OSTEOCHONDRODYSPLASIAS

Thanatophoric dysplasia

This is the most common lethal skeletal dysplasia with a birth prevalence of about 1 in 10 000. The term derives from the Greek, meaning death-bearing and the characteristic features are severe shortening of the limbs, narrow thorax, normal trunk length and large head with prominent forehead. In type I, which is sporadic, the femurs are curved (telephone receiver) and in type II, which is autosomal recessive, the femurs are straight but the skull is cloverleaf-shaped.

Achondrogenesis

This is a lethal skeletal dysplasia with a birth prevalence of about 1 in 40 000. The characteristic features are severe shortening of the limbs, narrow thorax, short trunk and large head. In achondrogenesis type I, which is autosomal recessive, there is poor mineralization of both the skull and vertebral bodies as well as rib fractures. In type II, which is sporadic (new autosomal dominant mutations), there is hypomineralization of the vertebral bodies but normal mineralization of the skull, and there are no rib fractures.

Osteogenesis imperfecta

Osteogenesis imperfecta is a genetically heterogeneous group of disorders presenting with fragility of bones, blue sclerae, loose joints and growth deficiency. The underlying defect is a dominant negative mutation affecting COL1A1 or COL1A2 alleles, which encode the proA1(I) and proa2(I) chains of type I collagen, a protein of paramount importance for normal skin and bone development. The mutations result in the production of abnormal quantity (OI type I) or quality (types II, III and IV) of collagen.

There are four clinical subtypes. In type I, which is an autosomal dominant condition with a birth prevalence of about 1 in 30 000, affected individuals have fragile bones, blue sclerae and progressive deafness, but life expectancy is normal. Prenatal diagnosis is available by DNA analysis. Ultrasonography in the second and third trimesters may demonstrate fractures of long bones.

In type II, which is a lethal disorder with a birth prevalence of about 1 in 60 000, most cases represent new dominant mutations (recurrence is about 6%). The disorder is characterized by early prenatal onset of severe bone shortening and bowing due to multiple fractures affecting all long bones and ribs, and poor mineralization of the skull.

Type III is a progressively deforming condition characterized by multiple fractures, usually present at birth, resulting in scoliosis and very short stature. Both autosomal dominant and recessive modes of inheritance have been reported.

Type IV is an autosomal dominant condition with variable expressivity. Severely affected individuals may have deformities of the long bones due to fractures. Prenatal diagnosis of types III and IV can be made by chorion villous sampling and DNA analysis, or by demonstration of abnormal collagen production in cultured fibroblasts.

Hypophosphatasia

This lethal, autosomal recessive condition, with a birth prevalence of about 1 in 100 000, is characterized by severe shortening of the long bones, small thorax, hypomineralization of the skull and long bones. There is absence of liver and bone isoenzymes of alkaline phosphatase, and first-trimester diagnosis is made by measurement of alkaline phosphatase isoenzymes in chorion villous samples. The diagnosis can also be made by DNA studies.

Achondroplasia

This autosomal dominant syndrome has a birth prevalence of about 1 in 26 000, but the majority of cases represent new mutations. The characteristic features of heterozygous achondroplasia include short limbs, lumbar lordosis, short hands and fingers, macrocephaly with frontal bossing and depressed nasal bridge. Intelligence and life expectancy are normal. Prenatally, limb shortening usually becomes apparent only after 22 weeks of gestation. In the homozygous state, which is a lethal condition, short limbs are associated with a narrow thorax. Achondroplasia is due to a specific mutation within the fibroblast growth factor receptor type 3 gene (FGFR3) and can now be diagnosed by DNA analysis of fetal blood or amniotic fluid obtained in cases of suspicious sonographic findings. In cases where both parents have achondroplasia, there is a 25% chance that the fetus is affected by the lethal type and the diagnosis can be made by first-trimester chorion villous sampling.

Campomelic dysplasia

This lethal, autosomal recessive syndrome with a birth prevalence of 1 in 200 000 is characterized by shortening and bowing of the long bones of the legs, narrow chest, hypoplastic scapulae, and large calvarium with disproportionately small face. Some of the affected genetically male individuals show a female phenotype. Patients usually die in the neonatal period from pulmonary hypoplasia.

Jarcho–Levin syndrome

This is a heterogeneous disorder, characterized by vertebral and rib abnormalities (misalignment of the cervical spine and ribs). An autosomal recessive type is characterized by a constricted short thorax and respiratory death in infancy. Another autosomal recessive and an autosomal dominant type are associated with a short stature and are compatible with survival to adult life but with some degree of physical disability.

Asphyxiating thoracic dysplasia (Jeune syndrome)

This is an autosomal recessive condition with a birth prevalence of about 1 in 70 000. The characteristic features are narrow chest and rhizomelic limb shortening. There is a variable phenotypic expression and, consequently, the prognosis varies from neonatal death, due to pulmonary hypoplasia, to normal survival. Limb shortening is mild to moderate and this may not become apparent until after 24 weeks of gestation.

Chondroectodermal dysplasia (Ellis–Van Creveld syndrome)

This rare, autosomal recessive condition is characterized by acromelic and mesomelic shortness of limbs, postaxial polydactyly, small chest, ectodermal dysplasia, and congenital heart defects in more than 50% of cases.

Short limb polydactyly syndromes

This group of lethal disorders is characterized by short limbs, narrow thorax and postaxial polydactyly. Associated anomalies are frequently found, including congenital heart disease, polycystic kidneys, and intestinal atresia. Four different types have been recognized. Type I (Saldino–Noonan) has narrow metaphyses; type II (Majewski) has cleft lip and palate and disproportionally shortened tibiae; type III (Naumoff) has wide metaphyses with spurs; type IV (Beemer–Langer) is characterized by median cleft lip, small chest with extremely short ribs, protuberant abdomen with umbilical hernia and ambiguous genitalia in some 46,XY individuals.

Diastrophic dysplasia

This autosomal recessive condition is characterized by severe shortening and bowing of all long bones, talipes equinovarus, hand deformities with abducted position of the thumbs ('hitchhiker thumb'), multiple joint flexion contractures and scoliosis. There is a wide spectrum in phenotypic expression and some cases may not be diagnosable *in utero*. This disease is not lethal and neurodevelopment is normal.

LIMB DEFICIENCY OR CONGENITAL AMPUTATIONS

Absence of an extremity or a segment of an extremity is referred to as 'limb deficiency' or 'congenital amputation'. The prevalence of limb reduction deformities is about 1 per 20 000 births. In about 50% of cases, there are simple transverse reduction deficiencies of one forearm or hand without associated anomalies. In the other 50% of cases, there are multiple reduction deficiencies and, in 25% of these, there are additional anomalies of the internal organs or craniofacial structures. In general, limb deficiency of the upper extremity is an isolated anomaly, whereas congenital amputation of the leg or bilateral amputations or reductions of all limbs are usually part of a genetic syndrome.

Isolated amputation of an extremity can be due to amniotic band syndrome, exposure to a teratogen or a vascular accident. There is an association between chorion villous sampling before 10 weeks of gestation and transverse limb defects. Syndromes associated with limb deficiencies include the aglossia–adactylia syndrome (transverse amputations of the limbs ranging from absent digits to severe deficiencies of all four extremities, micrognathia, and vestigial tongue or ankylosis of the tongue to the hard palate, the floor of the mouth or the lips), and the Moebius sequence (facial anomalies attributed to paralysis of the 6th and 7th cranial nerves, leading to micrognathia and ptosis with upper limb defects, ranging from transverse amputations to absent digits). Both syndromes are sporadic.

Limb reduction defects associated with other anomalies include the CHILD syndrome (congenital hemidysplasia with ichthyosiform erythroderma and limb defects). This is characterized by strict demarcation of the skin lesions to one side of the mid-line and limb deficiencies, which are unilateral, varying from hypoplasia of phalanges to complete absence of an extremity. The condition is also associated with heart defects and unilateral hydronephrosis or renal agenesis.

In phocomelia, the extremities resemble those of a seal. Typically, the hands and feet are present (these may be normal or abnormal), but the intervening arms and legs are absent. Phocomelia can also be caused by exposure to thalidomide, but this is only of historical interest. Three syndromes must be considered in the differential diagnosis of phocomelia: Roberts syndrome (autosomal recessive disorder characterized by the association of tetraphocomelia and facial clefting defects or hypoplastic nasal alae), some varieties of thrombocytopenia with absent radius (TAR syndrome) and Grebe syndrome (autosomal recessive condition, described in the inbred Indian tribes of Brazil, characterized by marked hypomelia of upper and lower limbs, increasing in severity from proximal to distal segments – in contrast to Roberts syndrome, the lower limbs are more affected than the upper extremities).

Congenital short femur has been classified into five groups: type I, simple hypoplasia of the femur; type II, short femur with angulated shaft; type III, short femur with coxa vara (the most common); type IV, absent or defective proximal femur; and type V, absent or rudimentary femur. One or both femurs can be affected but the right femur is more frequently involved. Femoral hypoplasia–unusual facies syndrome, which is sporadic, consists of bilateral femoral hypoplasia and facial defects, including short nose with broad tip, long philtrum, micrognathia and cleft palate.

If the defect is unilateral, it may correspond to the femur–fibula–ulna or femur–tibia–radius complex. These two syndromes have different implications for genetic counselling; the former is non-familial, while the second has a strong genetic component.

SPLIT HAND AND FOOT SYNDROME

The term 'split hand and foot' syndrome refers to a group of disorders characterized by splitting of the hand and foot into two parts; other terms include lobster-claw deformity and ectrodactyly. The conditions are classified into typical and atypical varieties. The typical variety (found in 1 per 90 000 births and usually inherited with an autosomal dominant pattern) consists of absence of both the finger and the metacarpal bone, resulting in a deep V-shaped central defect that clearly divides the hand into an ulnar and a radial part. The atypical variety (found in 1 per 150 000 births) is characterized by a much wider cleft formed by a defect of the metacarpals and the middle fingers; the cleft is U-shaped and wide, with only the thumb and small finger remaining.

Split hand and foot deformities can occur as isolated anomalies, but more commonly they are part of a more complex syndrome. Ectrodactyly–ectodermal dysplasia–cleft lip/palate syndrome (EEC syndrome), which is autosomal dominant, involves the four extremities with more severe deformities of the hands; the spectrum of ectodermal defects is wide, including dry skin, sparse hair, dental defects and defects of the tear duct. Other syndromes include split foot and triphalangeal thumb, split foot and hand and central polydactyly, Karsch–Neugebauer syndrome (split hand/foot with congenital nystagmus), acrorenal syndrome and mandibulofacial dysostosis (Fontaine syndrome).

CLUBHANDS

Clubhand deformities are classified into two main categories: radial and ulnar. Radial clubhand includes a wide spectrum of disorders that encompass absent thumb, thumb hypoplasia, thin first metacarpal and absent radius. Ulnar clubhand, which is less common, ranges from mild deviations of the hand on the ulnar side of the forearm to complete absence of the ulna. While radial clubhand is frequently syndromatic, ulnar clubhand is usually an isolated anomaly.

Clubhand deformities are often found in association with chromosomal abnormalities (such as trisomy 18), hematological abnormalities (such as Fanconi's pancytopenia, TAR syndrome and Aase syndrome), or genetic syndromes with cardiac defects (such as Holt–Oram syndrome, or the Lewis upper limb–cardiovascular syndrome). Radial clubhand is also associated with congenital scoliosis. The three syndromes that should be considered part of the differential diagnosis include the VATER association (vertebral segmentation, ventricular septal defect, anal atresia, tracheoesophageal fistula, radial and renal defects, and single umbilical artery), Goldenhar syndrome and the Klippel–Feil syndrome.

POLYDACTYLY

Polydactyly is the presence of an additional digit, which may range from a fleshy nubbin to a complete digit with controlled flexion and extension. Postaxial polydactyly (the most common form) occurs on the ulnar side of the hand and fibular side of the foot. Preaxial polydactyly is present on the radial side of the hand and the tibial side of the foot. The majority of conditions are isolated with an autosomal dominant mode of inheritance. Some of them are part of a syndrome, usually an autosomal recessive one. Preaxial polydactyly, especially triphalangeal thumb, is most likely to be part of a multisystem syndrome. Central polydactyly, which consists of an extra digit (usually hidden between the long and the ring finger), is often bilateral and is associated with other hand and foot malformations; it is inherited with an autosomal mode of inheritance.

FETAL AKINESIA DEFORMATION SEQUENCE (FADS)

This is a heterogeneous group of conditions with a birth prevalence of about 1 in 3000. Neurological, muscular, connective tissue, and skeletal abnormalities result in multiple joint contractures, including bilateral talipes and fixed flexion or extension deformities of the hips, knees, elbows and wrists. This sequence includes congenital lethal arthrogryposis, multiple pterygium and Pena–Shokeir syndromes. The deformities are usually symmetric and, in most cases, all four limbs are involved. The severity of the deformities increases distally in the involved limb, with the hands and feet typically being the most severely affected. The condition is commonly associated with polyhydramnios (usually after 25 weeks), narrow chest, micrognathia and nuchal edema (or increased nuchal translucency at 10–14 weeks).

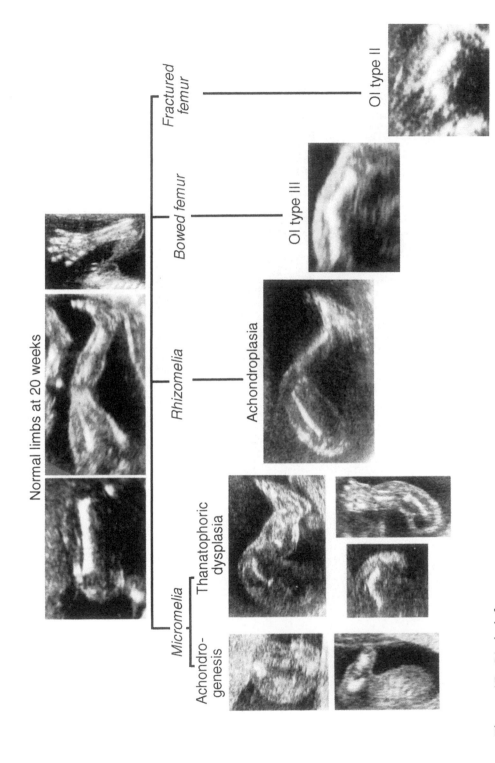

Figure 17 Limb defects

Normal thorax

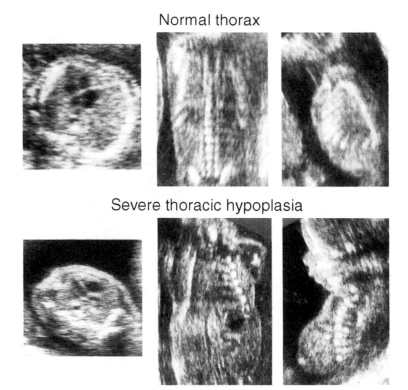

Severe thoracic hypoplasia

Figure 18 Thoracic defects

10

Features of chromosomal defects

Kypros Nicolaides and Rosalinde Snijders

PHENOTYPIC EXPRESSION

The commonest chromosomal defects are trisomies 21, 18 or 13, Turner syndrome (45,X), 47,XXX, 47,XXY, 47,XYY and triploidy. In the first trimester, a common feature of many chromosomal defects is increased nuchal translucency thickness. In later pregnancy, each chromosomal defect has its own syndromal pattern of abnormalities.

Trisomy 21

Trisomy 21 is associated with a tendency towards brachycephaly, mild ventriculomegaly, flattening of the face, nuchal edema, atrioventricular septal defects, duodenal atresia and echogenic bowel, mild hydronephrosis, shortening of the limbs, sandal gap and clinodactyly or mid-phalanx hypoplasia of the fifth finger.

Trisomy 18

Trisomy 18 is associated with strawberry-shaped head, choroid plexus cysts, absent corpus callosum, Dandy–Walker complex, facial cleft, micrognathia, nuchal edema, heart defects, diaphragmatic hernia, esophageal atresia, exomphalos, renal defects, myelomeningocele, growth retardation and shortening of the limbs, radial aplasia, overlapping fingers and talipes or rocker bottom feet.

Trisomy 13

In trisomy 13, common defects include holoprosencephaly and associated facial abnormalities, microcephaly, cardiac and renal abnormalities (often enlarged and echogenic kidneys), exomphalos and postaxial polydactyly.

Triploidy

Triploidy, where the extra set of chromosomes is paternally derived, is associated with a molar placenta and the pregnancy rarely persists beyond 20 weeks. When there is a double maternal chromosome contribution, the pregnancy may persist into the third trimester. The placenta is of normal consistency and the fetus demonstrates severe asymmetrical growth retardation. Commonly, there is mild ventriculomegaly, micrognathia, cardiac abnormalities, myelomeningocoele, syndactyly, and 'hitch-hiker' toe deformity.

Turner syndrome

There are two types of this syndrome, the lethal and non-lethal types. The rate of intrauterine lethality between 12 and 40 weeks is about 75%. The lethal type of Turner syndrome presents with large nuchal cystic hygromata, generalized edema, mild pleural effusions and ascites, and cardiac abnormalities. The non-lethal type usually does not demonstrate any ultrasonographic abnormalities.

Sex chromosome abnormalities

The main sex chromosome abnormalities, other than Turner syndrome, are 47,XXX, 47,XXY and 47,XYY. These are not associated with an increased prevalence of sonographically detectable defects.

Types of abnormalities

Table 1 shows the common chromosomal abnormalities in the presence of various sonographically detected defects.

RISK FOR CHROMOSOMAL DEFECTS

Number of defects

Ultrasound studies have demonstrated that major chromosomal defects are often associated with multiple fetal abnormalities. The overall risk for chromosomal defects increases with the total number of abnormalities that are identified. It is therefore recommended that, when an abnormality/marker is detected at routine ultrasound examination, a thorough check is made for the other features of the chromosomal defect(s) known to be associated with that marker; should additional abnormalities be identified, the risk is dramatically increased (Table 2, see p. 102).

Table 1 Common chromosomal abnormalities in fetuses with sonographic defects

	Trisomy 21	Trisomy 18	Trisomy 13	Triploidy	Turner
Skull/brain					
Strawberry-shaped head	−	+	−	−	−
Brachycephaly	+	+	+	−	+
Microcephaly	−	−	+	−	+
Ventriculomegaly	+	+	−	+	−
Holoprosencephaly	−	−	+	−	−
Choroid plexus cysts	+	+	−	−	−
Absent corpus callosum	−	+	−	−	−
Posterior fossa cyst	+	+	+	−	−
Enlarged cisterna magna	+	+	+	−	−
Face/neck					
Facial cleft	−	+	+	−	−
Micrognathia	−	+	−	+	−
Nuchal edema	+	+	+	−	−
Cystic hygromata	−	−	−	−	+
Chest					
Diaphragmatic hernia	−	+	+	−	−
Cardiac abnormality	+	+	+	+	+
Abdomen					
Exomphalos	−	+	+	−	−
Duodenal atresia	+	−	−	−	−
Collapsed stomach	+	+	−	−	−
Mild hydronephrosis	+	+	+	−	+
Other renal abnormalities	+	+	+	+	−
Other					
Hydrops	+	−	−	−	+
Small for gestational age	−	+	−	+	+
Relatively short femur	+	+	−	+	+
Clinodactyly	+	−	−	−	−
Overlapping fingers	−	+	−	−	−
Polydactyly	−	−	+	−	−
Syndactyly	−	−	−	+	−
Talipes	−	+	+	+	−

Table 2 Incidence of chromosomal defects in relation to number of sonographically detected abnormalities (Nicolaides *et al.*, *Lancet* 1992;340:704–7)

Abnormalities	n	Chromosomal defects
1	1128	2%
2	490	11%
3	220	32%
4	115	52%
5	53	66%
6	40	63%
7	16	69%
≥ 8	24	92%

Major defects

If the 18–23-week scan demonstrates major defects, it is advisable to offer fetal karyotyping even if these defects are apparently isolated. The prevalence of these defects is low and therefore the cost implications are small. If the defects are either lethal or they are associated with severe handicap, fetal karyotyping constitutes one of a series of investigations to determine the possible cause and therefore the risk of recurrence. Examples of these defects include hydrocephalus, holoprosencephaly, multicystic renal dysplasia and severe hydrops. In the case of isolated neural tube defects, there is controversy as to whether the risk for chromosomal defects is increased. Similarly, for skeletal dysplasias where the likely diagnosis is obvious by ultrasonography, it would probably be unnecessary to perform karyotyping. If the defect is potentially correctable by intrauterine or postnatal surgery, it may be logical to exclude an underlying chromosomal abnormality, especially because for many of these conditions the usual abnormality is trisomy 18 or 13. Examples include facial cleft, diaphragmatic hernia, esophageal atresia, exomphalos and many of the cardiac defects. In the case of isolated gastroschisis or small bowel obstruction, there is no evidence of increased risk of trisomies.

Minor defects or markers

For apparently isolated abnormalities, there are large differences in the reported incidence of associated chromosomal defects. It is therefore uncertain whether, in such cases, karyotyping should be undertaken, especially for those abnormalities that have a high prevalence in the general population and for which the prognosis in the absence of a chromosomal defect is good. Since the incidence of chromosomal defects is associated with maternal age, it is possible that the wide range of results reported in the various studies is the mere consequence of differences in the maternal age distribution of the populations examined. In addition, since chromosomal abnormalities are associated with a high rate of intrauterine death, differences may arise from the fact that studies were undertaken at different stages of pregnancy. For example, to determine whether apparently isolated choroid plexus cysts at 20 weeks of gestation are associated with an increased risk for trisomy 18, it is essential to know the incidence of trisomy 18 at 20 weeks, based on the maternal age distribution of the population that is examined. Therefore, we propose that, in the calculation of risks for chromosomal defects, it is necessary to take into account ultrasound findings as well as the maternal age and the gestational age at the time of the scan (see Appendix I, p. 125).

Association with maternal age and gestation

The risk for trisomies increases with maternal age and decreases with gestation; the rate of intrauterine lethality between 12 weeks and 40 weeks is about 30% for trisomy 21, and 80% for trisomies 18 and 13 (Appendix I). Turner syndrome is usually due to loss of the paternal X chromosome and, consequently, the frequency of conception of 45,X embryos, unlike that of trisomies, is unrelated to maternal age. The prevalence is about 1 per 1500 at 12 weeks, 1 per 3000 at 20 weeks and 1 per 4000 at 40 weeks. For the other sex chromosome abnormalities (47,XXX, 47,XXY and 47,XYY), there is no significant change with maternal age and, since the rate of intrauterine lethality is not higher than in chromosomally normal fetuses, the overall prevalence (about 1 per 500) does not decrease with gestation. Polyploidy affects about 2% of recognized conceptions but it is highly lethal and it is very rarely observed in live births; the prevalence at 12 and 20 weeks is about 1 per 2000 and 1 per 250 000, respectively.

Type of defect

If there are minor defects, the risk for trisomy 21 is calculated by multiplying the background (maternal age- and gestation-related risk) by a factor depending on the specific defect. For the following conditions, there are sufficient data in the literature to estimate the risk factors.

Nuchal edema or fold more than 6 mm   This is the second-trimester form of nuchal translucency. It is found in about 0.5% of fetuses and it may be of no pathological significance. However, it is sometimes associated with chromosomal defects, cardiac anomalies, infection or genetic syndromes. For isolated nuchal edema, the risk for trisomy 21 may be ten-times the background risk.

Hyperechogenic bowel   This is found in about 0.5% of fetuses and is usually of no pathological significance. The commonest cause is intra-amniotic bleeding, but occasionally it may be a marker of cystic fibrosis or chromosomal defects. For isolated hyperechogenic bowel, the risk for trisomy 21 may be seven-times the background risk.

Short femur   If the femur is below the 5th centile and all other measurements are normal, the baby is likely to be normal but rather short. Rarely, this is a sign of dwarfism. Occasionally, it may be a marker of chromosomal defects. On the basis of existing studies, short femur is found four-times as commonly in trisomy 21 fetuses compared to normal fetuses. However, there is some evidence that isolated short femur may not be more common in trisomic than normal fetuses.

Echogenic foci in the heart   These are found in about 4% of pregnancies and they are usually of no pathological significance. However, they are sometimes associated with cardiac defects and chromosomal abnormalities. For isolated hyperechogenic foci, the risk for trisomy 21 may be four-times the background risk.

Choroid plexus cysts   These are found in about 1–2% of pregnancies and they are usually of no pathological significance. When other defects are present, there is a high risk of chromosomal defects, usually trisomy 18 but occasionally trisomy 21. For isolated choroid plexus cysts, the risk for trisomy 18 and trisomy 21 is 1.5-times the background risk.

Mild hydronephrosis   This is found in about 1–2% of pregnancies and is usually of no pathological significance. When other abnormalities are present, there is a high risk of chromosomal defects, usually trisomy 21. For isolated mild hydronephrosis, the risk for trisomy 21 is 1.5-times the background risk.

11

Fetal tumors

Israel Meizner

INTRODUCTION

Fetal tumors are rare, but they have important implications for the health of both the fetus and the mother. The natural history and prognosis of most fetal tumors are well known. Once a fetal tumor has been detected, close surveillance by a multidisciplinary team of doctors is mandatory, with anticipation and early recognition of problems during pregnancy, labor and immediate postnatal life. When the sonographic diagnosis is uncertain, fetal tissue biopsy may be necessary to obtain a histological diagnosis. In rare cases, intrauterine treatment may be possible. Some fetal tumors may be malignant and could metastasize to other fetal organs and the placenta; maternal metastases in such cases are unknown. In contrast, on rare occasions, maternal malignancies (melanoma, leukemia and breast cancer) can metastasize to the placenta; in about half of the cases with placental metastases, mostly with malignant melanoma, the tumor can metastasize to fetal viscera.

Etiology and mechanisms of carcinogenesis

Developmental errors during embryonic and fetal maturation may result in embryonic tumors. One hypothesis is that more cells are produced than are required for the formation of an organ or tissue and the origins of embryonic tumors rest in developmental errors in these surplus embryonic rudiments. Embryonic tumors developing after infancy are explained by the persistence of cell rests or developmental vestiges. Developmentally anomalous tissue (such as hamartomas and dysgenic gonads) is a source of neoplasms in older children and adults. When any of this developmentally abnormal tissue is present at birth, it is inferred that the cells failed to mature, migrate or differentiate properly during intrauterine life.

Neoplastic transformation of cells in tissue culture and *in vivo* carcinogenesis are dynamic, multistep and complex processes that can be separated artificially into three phases: initiation, promotion and progression. These phases may be applied to the natural history of virtually all human tumors, including embryonic ones. *Initiation* is the result of exposure of cells or tissues to an appropriate dose of a carcinogen; an initiated cell is permanently damaged and has a malignant potential. The initiated cells can persist for months or years before becoming malignant. During the *promotion* phase, initiated cells clonally expand. Promotion may be modulated or reversed by a variety of environmental conditions. In the last phase, *progression*, the transformed cells develop into a tumor, ultimately with metastasis. Embryonic tumors can, therefore, be regarded as defects in the integrated control of cell differentiation and proliferation. A genetic model of carcinogenesis has also been introduced in an attempt to clarify the pathogenesis and behavioral peculiarities of certain embryonic tumors. According to this hypothesis, embryonal neoplasms arise as a result of two mutational events in the genome. The first mutation is prezygotic in familial cases and postzygotic in non-familial; the second mutation is always postzygotic.

Benignity of fetal and infantile neoplasms

Some neonatal and infantile tumors have a benign clinical behavior despite histological evidence of malignancy. Examples include congenital neuroblastomas and hepato-blastomas in the first year of life, and congenital and infantile fibromatosis, and sacrococcygeal teratomas in the first few months of life. The factors responsible for this 'oncogenic period of grace', which starts *in utero* and extends through the first few months of extrauterine life, are uncertain.

Association of neoplasia and congenital malformations

The concept that teratogenesis and oncogenesis have shared mechanisms is well docu-mented by numerous examples. Probably, there is simultaneous or sequential cellular and tissue reaction to specific injurious agents. The degree of cytodifferentiation, the metabolic or immunological state of the embryo or fetus, and the length of time of exposure to the agent will determine whether the effect is teratogenic, oncogenic, both, or neither. Many biological, chemical and physical agents known to be teratogenic to the fetus or embryo are carcinogenic postnatally. Alternatively, a teratogenic event during intrauterine life may predispose the fetus to an oncogenic event later in life. This would explain neoplastic transformation occurring in hamar-tomas, developmental vestiges, heterotopias and dysgenetic tissues. It is postulated that the anomalous tissues harbor latent oncogenes which, under certain environmental conditions, are activated, resulting in malignant transformation of a tumor.

Classification

A formal classification of fetal tumors does not exist. Apart from distinguishing solid from cystic lesions, probably the best classification should be by location. The main compartments of fetal tumors are the head and brain, face and neck, thorax (including the heart), abdomen and retroperitoneum, extremities, genitalia, sacrococcygeal region, and skin.

Prenatal diagnosis

The approach for prenatal diagnosis of fetal tumors should be based on three sets of ultrasound signs: general signs, organ-specific signs and tumor-specific signs. The *general sonographic features*, that should raise the suspicion of an underlying fetal tumor, include:

(1) Absence or disruption of contour, shape, location, sonographic texture or size, of a normal anatomic structure;

(2) Presence of an abnormal structure or abnormal biometry;

(3) Abnormality in fetal movement;

(4) Polyhydramnios; and

(5) Hydrops fetalis.

Polyhydramnios is particularly important, because almost 50% of fetal tumors are accompanied by this finding. The underlying mechanisms include interference with swallowing (such as thyroid goiter or myoblastoma), mechanical obstruction (such as gastrointestinal tumors), excessive production of amniotic fluid (such as sacrococcygeal teratoma), and decreased resorption by lung tissue in lung pathology. Intracranial tumors are also commonly associated with polyhydramnios and the mechanism may be neurogenic lack of swallowing or inappropriate polyuria.

Tumor-specific signs include pathological changes within the tumor mass (calcifications, liquefaction, organ edema, internal bleeding, neovascularization and rapid changes in size and texture). *Organ-specific signs* are rare, but in some cases they are highly suggestive of the condition (such as cardiomegaly with a huge solid or cystic mass occupying the entire heart, suggesting intrapericardial teratoma).

In some cases, normal and abnormal sonographic findings may mimic fetal tumors. Examples may vary from severe cases of bladder exstrophy (where the protruding bladder mass appears as a solid tumor-like structure), to rare cases of fetal scrotal inguinal hernia (where bowel loops occupy the scrotum, appearing as huge masses).

Prognosis

Apart from intracranial tumors (where the prognosis is generally poor), the prognosis for tumors in other locations is variable and depends on the size of the tumor (with resultant compression of adjacent organs), degree of vascularization (with the risk of causing heart failure and hydrops), and associated polyhydramnios (with the risk of preterm delivery).

INTRACRANIAL TUMORS

Intracranial tumors include teratomas, epidermoid, dermoid, germinoma, medulloblastoma, meningeal sarcoma, lipoma of the corpus callosum, oligodendroglioma, gangliocytoma, and glioblastoma, choroid plexus papilloma, tuberous sclerosis (Bourneville's disease), neurofibromatosis (Von Recklinghausen's disease), and systemic angiomatosis of the central nervous system and eye (Von Hippel–Lindau's disease).

Prevalence

Brain tumors are exceedingly rare in children, and only about 5% arise during fetal life; teratoma is the most frequently reported.

Etiology

Embryonic tumors are thought to derive from embryologically displaced cells. Brain tumors have been produced in animals by the use of chemical and viral teratogens. The relevance of these experiments to human brain neoplasms is unclear.

Diagnosis

A brain tumor should be suspected in the presence of mass-occupying lesions (cystic or solid areas), and a change in shape or size of the normal anatomic structures (such as shift in the mid-line). Cystic tumors and teratomas are usually characterized by complete loss of the normal intracranial architecture. In some cases, the lesion appears as a low echogenic structure, and it may be difficult to recognize. Hydrocephalus is frequently associated with brain tumors and may be the presenting sign. The ultrasound appearances of all intracranial tumors are similar and, therefore, precise histological diagnosis from a scan is almost impossible. Possible exceptions are lipomas (that have a typical hyperechogenic homogeneous appearance) and choroid plexus papillomas (that appear as an overgrowth of the choroid plexus). Identification of brain neoplasm associated with tuberous sclerosis, neurofibromatosis, and systemic angiomatosis of the central nervous system and eye can be attempted in patients at high risk; in most cases, however, antenatal sonography is negative, at least in the second trimester.

Prognosis

Prognosis depends on a number of factors, including the histological type and the size and location of the lesion. Congenital intracranial teratomas are usually fatal. The limited experience with the other neoplasms in prenatal diagnosis precludes the formulation of prognostic considerations.

TUMORS OF THE FACE AND NECK

Epignathus

This is a very rare teratoma arising from the oral cavity or pharynx. Most cases of epignathus arise from the sphenoid bone. Some arise from the hard and soft palate, the pharynx, the tongue and jaw. From their sites of origin, the tumors grow into the oral or nasal cavity or intracranially. The tumors, which are usually benign, consist of tissues derived from any of the three germinal layers; most of them contain adipose tissue, cartilage, bone, and nervous tissue. Prenatal diagnosis is suggested by the demonstration of a solid tumor arising from the oral cavity; calcifications and cystic components may also be present. Differential diagnosis includes neck teratomas, encephaloceles, and other tumors of the facial structures. Polyhydramnios (due to pharyngeal compression) is usually present. A careful examination of the brain is important because the tumor may grow intracranially. The outlook depends on the size of the lesion and the involvement of vital structures. Lesions detected antenatally have been very large. Polyhydramnios has been associated with poor prognosis. The major cause of neonatal death is asphyxia due to airway obstruction. Surgical resection with a normal postoperative course is possible.

Myoblastoma

This is a very rare benign tumor, which usually arises from the oral cavity. The tumor occurs in females exclusively and it may be the consequence of excessive production of estrogens by the fetal ovaries under human chorionic gonadotropin stimulation. The ultrasound features are those of a large solid mass protruding from the fetal mouth. Vascular connections between the tumor and the floor of the oral cavity may be demonstrated using color Doppler ultrasound. Polyhydramnios (due to pharyngeal compression) is common.

Cervical teratoma

This is a rare tumor. Ultrasound features include a unilateral and well-demarcated partly solid and cystic, or multiloculated mass, calcifications (in about 50% of cases), and polyhydramnios (in about 30% of cases due to esophageal obstruction). The prognosis is very poor and the intrauterine or neonatal mortality rate (due to airway obstruction) is about 80%. Survival after surgery is more than 80% but, since these tumors tend to be large, extensive neck dissection and multiple additional procedures are necessary to achieve complete resection of the tumor with acceptable functional and cosmetic results.

Goiter

Fetal goiter (enlargement of the thyroid gland) can be associated with hyperthyroidism (the result of iodine excess or deficiency, intrauterine exposure to antithyroid drugs or congenital metabolic disorders of thyroid synthesis), hypothyroidism or an euthyroid state. Ultrasound diagnosis is based on the demonstration of a solid, anteriorly located symmetric mass, which may result in hyperextension of the fetal head. Polyhydramnios is common due to mechanical obstruction of the esophagus. The prognosis depends on the basic cause of the goiter. Most cases are in women with a history of thyroid disease. Fetal blood sampling can aid in determining fetal thyroid status, especially in women suffering from Grave's disease where a transplacental transfer of drugs or thyroid-stimulating antibodies may result in fetal goiter. Maternal therapy usually corrects fetal hyperthyroidism. Direct fetal therapy in cases of fetal hypothyroidism can be undertaken by amniocentesis or by cordocentesis and this can result in resolution of the fetal goiter.

TUMORS OF THE THORAX

Lung tumors

Fetal lung tumors have not been reported in the literature. Other lesions, which are malformations, and which may appear as solid masses in the thorax, include cystic adenoid malformation of lung and extralobar lung sequestration.

Mediastinal tumors

Mediastinal tumors (which include neuroblastoma and hemangioma) may cause mediastinal shift, lung hypoplasia, hydrops and polyhydramnios (due to esophageal compression).

Rhabdomyoma (hamartoma) of the heart

Rhabdomyoma (which represents excessive growth of cardiac muscle) is the most common primary cardiac tumor in the fetus, neonate, and young child; the birth prevalence is 1 per 10 000. In 50% of cases, the tumor is associated with tuberous sclerosis (autosomal dominant condition with a high degree of penetrance and variable expressivity). The ultrasound features are those of a single or multiple echogenic masses impinging upon the cardiac cavities. The prognosis depends on the number, size and location of the tumors. The clinical spectrum varies from completely asymptomatic to severely ill. The mortality rate in infants operated on within the first year of life is about 30%. Up to 80% of the infants with tuberous sclerosis have seizures and mental retardation, which are the most serious long-term complications of the disease.

Intrapericardial teratoma

In the majority of cases, the tumor is located in the right side of the heart. It may reach a size that is 2–3 times that of the normal heart. The tumor may be cystic or pedunculated. Pericardial effusion is always present and results from rupture of cystic areas within the tumor, or from obstruction of cardiac and pericardial lymphatic veins. Cardiac tamponade and hydrops may develop and the prognosis is very poor.

TUMORS OF THE ABDOMEN AND RETROPERITONEUM

Hepatic tumors

Primary hepatic tumors (hemangioma, mesenchymal hamartoma, hepatoblastoma and adenoma) are extremely rare. All hepatic tumors may show the same sonographic features: either a defined lesion (cystic or solid) is present or hepatomegaly exists. Calcifications may appear, and both oligohydramnios and polyhydramnios have been observed. The other tumors are very rare and little is known about their natural history. Hemangiomata are histologically benign and they regress spontaneously after infancy. However, occasionally, they are associated with arteriovenous shunting, congestive heart failure and hydrops, resulting in intrauterine or neonatal death.

Neuroblastoma

This is one of the most common tumors of infancy and is found in about 1 per 20 000 births. Neuroblastoma arises from undifferentiated neural tissue of the adrenal medulla or sympathetic ganglia in the abdomen, thorax, pelvis, or head and neck. Usually, the lesion is isolated, but occasional metastasis before birth may occur. Sonographically, the tumor appears as a cystic, solid, or complex mass in the region of the adrenal gland (directly above the level of the kidney and under the diaphragm). Occasionally, calcifications are present. Tumors arising from the sympathetic ganglia may appear in the neck, chest, or in the abdomen. There may be associated polyhydramnios and fetal hydrops. The tumor can metastasize *in utero* (placenta, liver, or blood vessels). The prognosis is excellent if the diagnosis is made *in utero* or in the first year of life (survival more than 90%), but, for those diagnosed after the first year, survival is less than 20%.

Renal tumors

Mesoblastic nephroma (renal hamartoma) is the most frequent renal tumor, while Wilms' tumor (nephroblastoma) is extremely rare. The sonographic picture in both tumors is of a solitary mass replacing the normal architecture of the kidney, and, in most cases, there is associated polyhydramnios. Cystic areas may appear in both tumors. Mesoblastic nephromas are benign, and nephrectomy is curative in the majority of cases. Wilms' tumor is a genetically heterogeneous group of malignant tumors and up to 60% of affected cases are associated with genetic syndromes (such as Beckwith–Wiedemann syndrome). Treatment of the tumor requires surgery, chemotherapy and sometimes radiotherapy.

TUMORS OF THE EXTREMITIES

Tumors of the extremities include:

(1) Vascular hamartosis; a malformation in which newly formed vessels proliferate;

(2) Hemangioma, a combined lesion of both skin and internal organs. The Klippel–Weber–Trenaunay syndrome should be considered in the differential diagnosis. The hemangiomas may vary in size and location. Some authors do not consider them to be true tumors, but rather suspect them to represent vascular malformations;

(3) Lymphangioma, a cavernous lymphangioma, which involves the lymphatic vessels and is related to cystic hygroma;

(4) Sarcoma (mainly rhabdomyosarcoma); this should be distinguished from infantile myofibromatosis.

TUMORS OF THE SKIN

Malignant melanoma is a rare tumor capable of metastasizing into other organs including the fetal liver, lungs and placenta.

SACROCOCCYGEAL TERATOMA

The sacrococcygeal region is the most frequent site of teratomas of the fetus.

Prevalence

Sacrococcygeal teratoma is found in about 1 per 40 000 births. Females are four times more likely to be affected than males, but malignant change is more common in males.

Etiology

This tumor is thought to arise from totipotential cells in Hensen's node. A theory of 'twinning accident' with incomplete separation during embryogenesis has also been proposed. The condition is sporadic but some cases are familial, with autosomal dominant inheritance.

Diagnosis

Sacrococcygeal teratomas usually appear solid or mixed solid and cystic (multiple cysts are irregular in shape and size). Occasionally, the tumor is completely cystic, and more rarely completely solid. Most teratomas are extremely vascular, which is easily shown using color Doppler ultrasound. The tumors may be entirely external, partially internal and partly external, or mainly internal. Polyhydramnios is frequent, and this may be due to direct transudation into the amniotic fluid and due to fetal polyuria, secondary to the hyperdynamic circulation, which is the consequence of arteriovenous shunting. Similarly, high-output heart failure leading to hepatomegaly, placentomegaly and hydrops fetalis can occur.

Prognosis

Sacrococcygeal teratoma is associated with a high perinatal mortality (about 50%), mainly due to the preterm delivery (the consequence of polyhydramnios) of a hydropic infant requiring major neonatal surgery. Difficult surgery, especially with tumors that extend into the pelvis and abdomen, can result in nerve injury and incontinence. The tumor is invariably benign in the neonatal period but delayed surgery or incomplete excision can result in malignant transformation (about 10% before 2 months of age to about 80% by 4 months).

12

Hydrops fetalis

Hydrops is defined by abnormal accumulation of serous fluid in skin (edema) and body cavities (pericardial, pleural, or ascitic effusions).

Prevalence

Hydrops fetalis is found in about 1 per 2000 births.

Etiology

Hydrops is a non-specific finding in a wide variety of fetal and maternal disorders, including hematological, chromosomal, cardiovascular, renal, pulmonary, gastro-intestinal, hepatic and metabolic abnormalities, congenital infection, neoplasms and malformations of the placenta or umbilical cord (see Table on next page). Hydrops is classically divided into immune (due to maternal hemolytic antibodies) and non-immune (due to all other etiologies). With the widespread introduction of immuno-prophylaxis and the successful treatment of Rhesus disease by fetal blood transfusions, non-immune causes have become responsible for at least 75% of the cases, and make a greater contribution to perinatal mortality. While, in many instances, the underlying cause may be determined by maternal antibody and infection screening, fetal ultra-sound scanning, including echocardiography and Doppler studies, and fetal blood sampling, quite often the abnormality remains unexplained even after expert postmor-tem examination.

Prognosis

Although isolated ascites, both in fetuses and neonates, may be transitory, the spontane-ous resolution of hydrops has not been reported and the overall mortality for this condi-tion is about 80%.

Fetal therapy

Immune hydrops can be successfully treated by blood transfusions to the fetus. Such treatment often results in reversal of hydrops and the survival rate is about 80%. Fetal therapy can also successfully reverse some types of non-immune hydrops, such as fetal tachyarrhythmias (by transplacental or direct fetal administration of antiarrhythmic drugs), pleural effusions (by pleuro-amniotic shunting), urinary ascites (by vesico-amniotic or peritoneal-amniotic shunting), parvovirus B19 infection or severe fetomaternal hemorrhage (by fetal blood transfusions), diaphragmatic hernia, cystic adenomatoid malformation of the lungs and sacrococcygeal teratoma (by open or endoscopic fetal surgery), and the recipient fetus in twin-to-twin transfusion syndrome (by endoscopic laser coagulation of the communicating placental vessels).

Causes of fetal hydrops

Heart failure
Cardiac defects
Dysrhythmias
Myocarditis
Fetal anemia
Arteriovenous shunts
Mediastinal compression
Cardiomyopathy
Recipient in twin transfusion

Myocarditis
Coxsackie virus
Parvovirus B19

Anemia
Red cell isoimmunization
Parvovirus B19
Cytomegalovirus
Alpha-thalassemia
Fetomaternal hemorrhage
G-6-PD deficiency

Arteriovenous shunts
Fetal tumor
Vein of Galen aneurysm
Placental chorioangioma
Acardiac twin

Mediastinal compression
Skeletal dysplasias
Diaphragmatic hernia
Cystic adenomatoid malformation
Pulmonary sequestration
Laryngeal obstruction

Hypoproteinemia
Renal defects
Gastrointestinal defects
Hepatic infiltration

Hepatic infiltration
Fetal anemia
Fetal infection
Metabolic disorder

Fetal infection
Cytomegalovirus
Toxoplasmosis
Rubella
Syphylis
Hepatitis

Metabolic disorder
Mucopolysaccharidosis
Gaucher's disease
Hurler's syndrome
Gangliosidosis
Sialidosis

Neuromuscular
Fetal akinesia deformation sequence

Chromosomal
Trisomies 21, 18 or 13
Turner syndrome
Triploidy

13

Small for gestational age

Small-for-gestational-age fetuses are defined by the finding that the abdominal circumference is below the 5th centile for gestation. About 80% of such fetuses are constitutionally small, with no increased perinatal death or morbidity, 15% are growth-restricted due to reduced placental perfusion and 'uteroplacental insufficiency', and 5% are growth-restricted due to low growth potential, the result of genetic disease or environmental damage.

Ultrasound findings

The finding of a small abdominal circumference should stimulate the sonographer to consider four possible causes: wrong dates, normal small, abnormal small or starving small fetus. Accurate measurements of the head and abdominal circumference, femur length and transverse cerebellar diameter should be taken and their various ratios should be examined. Additionally, a detailed examination should be carried out for the detection of any defects or markers of chromosomal abnormalities (mainly triploidy and trisomy 18), and for assessment of amniotic fluid and fetal activity.

In cases of *wrong dates,* there may be a suggestive history (uncertain last menstrual period, irregular cycle, conception within 3 months of stopping the contraceptive pill or breast feeding), all measurements are symmetrically small, there are no obvious anatomical defects, and their amniotic fluid volume and fetal activity are normal. A repeat ultrasound examination in 2 weeks will demonstrate an increase in fetal measurements and the rate of growth is normal (the lines joining the measurements are parallel to the appropriate normal mean for gestation).

In *normal small fetuses,* the mother is usually small (the main determinant of fetal size is maternal size), and the ultrasound findings are similar to pregnancies with wrong dates. However, a repeat scan in 2 weeks may demonstrate a further deviation from normal in the various fetal measurements.

In *starving small fetuses*, the fetal measurements demonstrate asymmetry (the greatest deficit is observed in the abdominal circumference, then the femur length and finally the head circumference with the transverse cerebellar diameter being the least affected); there are no obvious fetal anatomical defects, the amniotic fluid and fetal movements are reduced, the placenta is often thickened with translucent areas (placental lakes) and there are abnormal Doppler waveforms in the uterine and/or umbilical arteries. In severe hypoxia, the fetal heart appears dilated and the bowel is hyperechogenic or mildly dilated.

In *abnormal small fetuses*, there may be anatomical defects suggestive of chromosomal abnormalities (in triploidy, there may be a molar placenta or, in the presence of a normal placenta, the fetus demonstrates severe asymmetrical growth restriction, mild ventriculomegaly, micrognathia, cardiac abnormalities, myelomeningocele, syndactyly, or 'hitch-hiker' toe deformity; trisomy is characterized by strawberry-shaped head, choroid plexus cysts, absent corpus callosum, enlarged cisterna magna, facial cleft, micrognathia, nuchal edema, heart defects, diaphragmatic hernia, esophageal atresia, exomphalos, renal defects, myelomeningocele, growth retardation and shortening of the limbs, radial aplasia, overlapping fingers and talipes or rocker bottom feet). The amniotic fluid may be normal, decreased or often increased. In congenital infection, growth restriction may be associated with features of hydrops and brain abnormalities (ventriculomegaly, microcephaly or cerebral calcifications).

Doppler ultrasound

Doppler ultrasound provides a non-invasive method for the study of fetal hemodynamics. Investigation of the uterine and umbilical arteries provides information on the perfusion of the uteroplacental and fetoplacental circulations, respectively, while Doppler studies of selected fetal organs are valuable in detecting the hemodynamic rearrangements that occur in response to fetal hypoxemia. In normal pregnancy, impedance to flow in the uterine artery decreases with gestation and this presumably reflects the trophoblastic invasion of the spiral arteries and their conversion into low resistance vessels. Similarly, there is a decrease in impedance to flow in the umbilical arteries due to progressive maturation of the placenta and increase in the number of tertiary stem villi.

In constitutionally small fetuses (*normal small*), Doppler studies of the placental and fetal circulations are normal. Similarly, in growth-restricted fetuses due to genetic disease (*abnormal small*), the results are often normal. In growth restriction due to placental insufficiency (*starving small*), there is increased impedance to flow in the uterine arteries (with the characteristic waveform of early diastolic notching) and umbilical arteries (high pulsatility index and, in severe cases, absence of reversal of end-diastolic frequencies). Histopathological studies have shown in this condition failure of the normal development of maternal placental arteries into low resistance vessels (and therefore reduced oxygen and nutrient supply to the intervillous space), and reduction in the number of placental terminal capillaries and small muscular arteries in the tertiary stem villi (and therefore impaired maternal–fetal transfer). Doppler studies of the fetal circulation demonstrate decrease in impedance to flow in the middle cerebral arteries and increase in impedance in the descending thoracic aorta and renal artery. These findings suggest that, in fetal hypoxemia, there is an increase in the blood supply to the brain and reduction in the perfusion of the kidneys, gastrointestinal tract and the lower extremities. Although knowledge of the factors governing circulatory readjustments and their mechanism of action is incomplete, it appears that partial pressures of oxygen and carbon dioxide play a role, presumably through their action on chemoreceptors. In severe fetal hypoxemia, there is decompensation in the cardiovascular system and right heart failure. This is manifested by the absence or reversal of forward flow during atrial contraction in the ductus venosus and this is a sign of impending fetal death.

Chromosomal defects

Although low birth weight is a common feature of many chromosomal abnormalities, the incidence of chromosomal defects in small-for-gestational-age neonates is less than 1–2%. However, data derived from postnatal studies underestimate the association between chromosomal abnormalities and growth restriction, since many pregnancies with chromosomally abnormal fetuses result in intrauterine death. Thus, in fetuses presenting with growth restriction in the second trimester, the incidence of chromosomal abnormalities is 10–20%. The chromosomal abnormalities associated with severe growth restriction are triploidy, trisomy 18 and deletion of the short arm of chromosome 4. The incidence of chromosomal defects is much higher in:

(1) Fetuses with multiple malformations than in those with no structural defects;

(2) The group with normal or increased amniotic fluid volume than in those with reduced or absent amniotic fluid; and,

(3) The group with normal waveforms from both uterine and umbilical arteries than in those with abnormal waveforms from either or both vessels.

A substantial proportion of the chromosomally abnormal fetuses demonstrates the asymmetry (high head to abdomen circumference ratio) thought to be typical for uteroplacental insufficiency; indeed the most severe form of asymmetrical growth restriction is found in fetuses with triploidy.

119

Growth restriction can also be caused by confined placental mosaicism. In this condition, which is found in about 1% of pregnancies, the fetal karyotype is normal but there are two different chromosomal complements in the placenta (one is usually normal and the other an autosomal trisomy). Placental mosaicism is also associated with uniparental disomy (inheritance of two homologous chromosomes from one parent), which often results in growth restriction.

14

Abnormalities of the amniotic fluid volume

Amniotic fluid is produced by fetal urination but, in the first 16 weeks of gestation, additional sources include the placenta, amniotic membranes, umbilical cord and fetal skin. Removal of amniotic fluid is by fetal swallowing. Ultrasonographically, the diagnosis of polyhydramnios or oligohydramnios is made when there is excessive or virtual absence of echo-free spaces around the fetus.

OLIGOHYDRAMNIOS/ANHYDRAMNIOS

Oligohydramnios means reduced amniotic fluid and anhydramnios means absence of amniotic fluid.

Prevalence

Oligohydramnios in the second trimester is found in about 1 per 500 pregnancies.

Etiology

Oligohydramnios in the second trimester is usually the result of preterm premature rupture of the membranes, uteroplacental insufficiency and urinary tract malformations (bilateral renal agenesis, multicystic or polycystic kidneys, or urethral obstruction).

Diagnosis

The diagnosis of oligohydramnios is usually made subjectively. Quantitative criteria include, first, the largest single pocket of amniotic fluid being 1 cm or less, or, second, amniotic fluid index (the sum of the vertical measurements of the largest pockets of amniotic fluid in the four quadrants of the uterus) of less than 5 cm. In the absence of the 'acoustic window' normally provided by the amniotic fluid, and the 'undesirable' postures often adopted by these fetuses, confident exclusion of fetal defects may be impossible. Nevertheless, the detection of a dilated bladder in urethral obstruction and enlarged echogenic or multicystic kidneys in renal disease should be relatively easy. The main difficulty is in the differential diagnosis of renal agenesis. In cases of preterm prelabor rupture of the membranes, detailed questioning of the mother may reveal a history of chronic leakage of amniotic fluid. Furthermore, in uteroplacental insufficiency, Doppler blood flow studies will often demonstrate high impedance to flow in the placental circulation and redistribution in the fetal circulation. In the remaining cases, intra-amniotic instillation of normal saline may help to improve ultrasonographic examination and lead to the diagnosis of fetal abnormalities like renal agenesis.

Prognosis

Bilateral renal agenesis, multicystic or polycystic kidneys are lethal abnormalities, usually in the neonatal period due to pulmonary hypoplasia. Preterm rupture of membranes at 20 weeks or earlier is associated with a poor prognosis; about 40% miscarry within 5 days of membrane rupture due to chorioamnionitis, and, in the remaining 60% of pregnancies, more than 50% of neonates die due to pulmonary hypoplasia. Uteroplacental insufficiency resulting in oligohydramnios at 18–23 weeks is very severe and the most likely outcome is intrauterine death.

POLYHYDRAMNIOS

Polyhydramnios means increased or excessive amniotic fluid volume.

Prevalence

Polyhydramnios in the second trimester is found in about 1 per 200 pregnancies.

Etiology

There are essentially two major causes of polyhydramnios: reduced fetal swallowing or absorption of amniotic fluid and increased fetal urination. Reduced fetal swallowing may be due to craniospinal defects (such as anencephaly), facial tumors, gastrointestinal obstruction (such as esophageal atresia, duodenal atresia and small bowel obstruction), compressive pulmonary disorders (such as pleural effusions, diaphragmatic hernia or cystic adenomatoid malformation of the lungs), narrow thoracic cage (due to skeletal dysplasias), and fetal akinesia deformation sequence (due to neuromuscular impairment of fetal swallowing). Increased fetal urination is observed in maternal diabetes mellitus and maternal uremia (increased glucose and urea cause osmotic diuresis), hyperdynamic fetal circulation due to fetal anemia (due to red cell isoimmunization or congenital infection) or fetal and placental tumors or cutaneous arteriovenous malformations (such as sacrococcygeal teratoma, placental chorioangioma), or twin-to-twin transfusion syndrome.

Diagnosis

The diagnosis of polyhydramnios is usually made subjectively. Quantitatively, polyhydramnios is defined as an amniotic fluid index (the sum of the vertical measurements of the largest pockets of amniotic fluid in the four quadrants of the uterus) of 20 cm or more. Alternatively, the vertical measurement of the largest single pocket of amniotic fluid free of fetal parts is used to classify polyhydramnios into mild (8–11 cm), moderate (12–15 cm) and severe (16 cm or more). Although 80% of cases with mild polyhydramnios are considered to be idiopathic, in the majority of cases with moderate or severe polyhydramnios there are maternal or fetal disorders. In most cases, polyhydramnios develops late in the second or in the third trimester of pregnancy. Acute polyhydramnios at 18–23 weeks is mainly seen in association with twin-to-twin transfusion syndrome. Testing for maternal diabetes, detailed sonographic examination for anomalies, and fetal karyotyping should constitute the cornerstones of the diagnostic protocol in the investigation of these cases.

Prenatal therapy

The aim is to reduce the risk of very premature delivery and the maternal discomfort that often accompanies severe polyhydramnios. Treatment will obviously depend on the diagnosis, and will include better glycemic control of maternal diabetes mellitus, antiarrhythmic medication for fetal hydrops due to dysrhythmias, thoracoamniotic shunting for fetal pulmonary cysts or pleural effusions. For the other cases, polyhydramnios may be treated by repeated amniocenteses every few days and drainage of large volumes of amniotic fluid. However, the procedure itself may precipitate premature labor. An alternative and effective method of treatment is maternal administration of indomethacin; however, this drug may cause fetal ductal constriction, and close monitoring by serial fetal echocardiographic studies is necessary. In twin-to-twin transfusion syndrome, presenting with acute polyhydramnios at 18–23 weeks of gestation, endoscopic laser occlusion of placental anastomoses or serial amniodrainage may be carried out.

Prognosis

This depends on the cause of polyhydramnios.

Appendix I: Risk of major trisomies in relation to maternal age and gestation

Table 1 Trisomy 21 (Snijders *et al. Ultrasound Obstet Gynecol* 1999;13:167–70)

Maternal age (years)	Gestational age					
	10 weeks	*12 weeks*	*14 weeks*	*16 weeks*	*20 weeks*	*40 weeks*
20	1/983	1/1068	1/1140	1/1200	1/1295	1/1527
25	1/870	1/946	1/1009	1/1062	1/1147	1/1352
30	1/576	1/626	1/668	1/703	1/759	1/895
31	1/500	1/543	1/580	1/610	1/658	1/776
32	1/424	1/461	1/492	1/518	1/559	1/659
33	1/352	1/383	1/409	1/430	1/464	1/547
34	1/287	1/312	1/333	1/350	1/378	1/446
35	1/229	1/249	1/266	1/280	1/302	1/356
36	1/180	1/196	1/209	1/220	1/238	1/280
37	1/140	1/152	1/163	1/171	1/185	1/218
38	1/108	1/117	1/125	1/131	1/142	1/167
39	1/82	1/89	1/95	1/100	1/108	1/128
40	1/62	1/68	1/72	1/76	1/82	1/97
41	1/47	1/51	1/54	1/57	1/62	1/73
42	1/35	1/38	1/41	1/43	1/46	1/55
43	1/26	1/29	1/30	1/32	1/35	1/41
44	1/20	1/21	1/23	1/24	1/26	1/30
45	1/15	1/16	1/17	1/18	1/19	1/23

Table 2   Trisomy 18 (Snijders *et al. Fetal Diag Ther* 1995;10:356–67)

Maternal age (years)	Gestational age					
	10 weeks	12 weeks	14 weeks	16 weeks	20 weeks	40 weeks
20	1/1993	1/2484	1/3015	1/3590	1/4897	1/18013
25	1/1765	1/2200	1/2670	1/3179	1/4336	1/15951
30	1/1168	1/1456	1/1766	1/2103	1/2869	1/10554
31	1/1014	1/1263	1/1533	1/1825	1/2490	1/9160
32	1/860	1/1072	1/1301	1/1549	1/2490	1/7775
33	1/715	1/891	1/1081	1/1287	1/1755	1/6458
34	1/582	1/725	1/880	1/1047	1/1429	1/5256
35	1/465	1/580	1/703	1/837	1/1142	1/4202
36	1/366	1/456	1/553	1/659	1/899	1/3307
37	1/284	1/354	1/430	1/512	1/698	1/2569
38	1/218	1/272	1/330	1/393	1/537	1/1974
39	1/167	1/208	1/252	1/300	1/409	1/1505
40	1/126	1/157	1/191	1/227	1/310	1/1139
41	1/95	1/118	1/144	1/171	1/233	1/858
42	1/71	1/89	1/108	1/128	1/175	1/644
43	1/53	1/66	1/81	1/96	1/131	1/481
44	1/40	1/50	1/60	1/72	1/98	1/359

Table 3   Trisomy 13 (Snijders *et al. Fetal Diag Ther* 1995;10:356–67)

Maternal age (years)	Gestational age					
	10 weeks	12 weeks	14 weeks	16 weeks	20 weeks	40 weeks
20	1/6347	1/7826	1/9389	1/11042	1/14656	1/42423
25	1/5621	1/6930	1/8314	1/9778	1/12978	1/37567
30	1/3719	1/4585	1/5501	1/6470	1/8587	1/24856
31	1/3228	1/3980	1/4774	1/5615	1/7453	1/21573
32	1/2740	1/3378	1/4052	1/4766	1/6326	1/18311
33	1/2275	1/2806	1/3366	1/3959	1/5254	1/15209
34	1/1852	1/2284	1/2740	1/3222	1/4277	1/12380
35	1/1481	1/1826	1/2190	1/2576	1/3419	1/9876
36	1/1165	1/1437	1/1724	1/2027	1/2691	1/7788
37	1/905	1/1116	1/1339	1/1575	1/2090	1/6050
38	1/696	1/858	1/1029	1/1210	1/1606	1/4650
39	1/530	1/654	1/784	1/922	1/1224	1/3544
40	1/401	1/495	1/594	1/698	1/927	1/2683
41	1/302	1/373	1/447	1/526	1/698	1/2020
42	1/227	1/280	1/335	1/395	1/524	1/1516
43	1/170	1/209	1/251	1/295	1/392	1/1134
44	1/127	1/156	1/187	1/220	1/292	1/846

Appendix II: Antenatal sonographic findings in skeletal dysplasias

Type of limb shortening

Rhizomelia
Thanatophoric dysplasia
Atelosteogenesis
Chondrodysplasia punctata (rhizomelic type)
Diastrophic dysplasia
Congenital short femur
Achondroplasia

Mesomelia
Mesomelic dysplasia
COVESDEM association
Acromelia
Ellis–Van Creveld syndrome

Micromelia
Achondrogenesis
Atelosteogenesis
Short-rib polydactyly syndrome (types I and III)
Diastrophic dysplasia
Fibrochondrogenesis
Osteogenesis imperfecta (type II)
Kniest dysplasia
Dyssegmental dysplasia

Altered thoracic dimensions

Long narrow thorax
Asphyxiating thoracic dysplasia
Ellis–Van Creveld syndrome
Metatropic dysplasia
Fibrochondrogenesis
Atelosteogenesis
Campomelic dysplasia
Jarcho–Levin syndrome
Achondrogenesis
Hypophosphatasia
Dyssegmental dysplasia
Cleidocranial dysplasia

Short thorax
Osteogenesis imperfecta (type II)
Kniest's dysplasia
Pena–Shokeir syndrome
Hypoplastic thorax
Short-rib polydactyly syndrome (types I and II)
Thanatophoric dysplasia
Cerebro-costo-mandibular syndrome
Cleidocranial dysostosis syndrome
Homozygous achondroplasia
Melnick–Needles syndrome (osteodysplasty)
Fibrochondrogenesis
Otopalatodigital syndrome (type II)

Hand and foot abnormalities

Postaxial polydactyly
Chondroectodermal dysplasia
Short rib-polydactyly syndrome (type I,
    type III)
Asphyxiating thoracic dysplasia
Otopalatodigital syndrome
Mesomelic dysplasia Werner type
    (associated with absence of thumbs)

Preaxial polydactyly
Chondroectodermal dysplasia
Short-rib polydactyly syndrome type II
Carpenter syndrome

Syndactyly
Poland syndrome
Carpenter syndrome
Aper syndrome
Otopalatodigital syndrome (type II)
Mesomelic dysplasia Werner type
TAR syndrome
Jarcho–Levin syndrome
Roberts syndrome

Brachydactyly
Mesomelic dysplasia Robinow type
Otopalatodigital syndrome

Hitch-hiker thumb
Diastrophic dysplasia

Clubfeet deformity
Diastrophic dysplasia
Osteogenesis imperfecta
Kniest dysplasia
Spondyloepiphyseal dysplasia congenita

Skull and face deformities

Large head
Achondroplasia
Achondrogenesis
Thanatophoric dysplasia
Osteogenesis imperfecta
Cleidocranial dysplasia
Hypophosphatasia
Campomelic syndrome
Short rib-polydactyly syndrome (type III)
Robinow mesomelic dysplasia
Otopalatodigital syndrome

Clover-leaf skull
Thanatophoric dysplasia (type II)
Campomelic syndrome

Other craniostenosis
Apert's syndrome
Carpenter syndrome
Hypophosphatasia

Congenital cataracts
Chondrodysplasia punctata

Cleft palate
Asphyxiating thoracic dysplasia
Kniest dysplasia
Diastrophic dysplasia
Spondyloepiphyseal syndrome
Campomelic syndrome
Jarcho–Levin syndrome
Chondroectodermal dysplasia
Short-rib polydactyly syndrome (type II)
Metatropic dysplasia
Dyssegmental dysplasia
Otopalatodigital syndrome (type II)
Roberts syndrome

Hypertelorism
Otopalatodigital syndrome
Arthrogryposis multiplex congenita
Larsen's syndrome
Roberts syndrome
Cleidocranial dysplasia
Achondroplasia
Campomelic dysplasia
Coffin syndrome
Klippel–Feil syndrome
Aper syndrome
Sprengel's deformity
Mesomelic dysplasia
Holt–Oram syndrome

Micrognathia
Campomelic dysplasia
Diastrophic dysplasia
Otopalatodigital syndrome
Achondrogenesis
Mesomelic dysplasia
Arthrogryposis multiplex congenita
Nager acrofacial dysostosis
Oromandibular limb hypogenesis
Atelosteogenesis

Appendix III: Fetal biometry at 14–40 weeks of gestation

The normal ranges for fetal biometry presented in this section were established from cross-sectional data on 1040 singleton pregnancies at 14–40 weeks of gestation (Snijders & Nicolaides, *Ultrasound Obstet Gynecol* 1994;4:34–48). The patients fulfilled the following criteria: (1) known last menstrual period with a cycle length of 26–30 days, (2) no fetal abnormalities and no pregnancy complications, (3) live birth at term, (4) birth weight above the 3rd and below the 97th centile for gestation (Yudkin *et al.*, *Early Hum Dev* 1987;15:45–52). For each 7-day interval from 14 to 40 weeks, 40 patients were included.

Measurements of biparietal diameter (BPD), occipito-frontal diameter (OFD), anterior and posterior cerebral ventricle diameter (Va and Vp), and hemisphere (H) were obtained from a transverse axial plane of the fetal head showing a central mid-line echo broken in the anterior third by the cavum septii pellucidi and demonstrating the anterior and posterior horns of the lateral ventricles. BPD and OFD were measured from the outer borders of the skull and head circumference (HC) was calculated [3.14 × (BPD+OFD)/2]. Va was the distance between the lateral wall of the anterior horn to the mid-line and Vp was the distance between the medial and lateral walls of the posterior horn. The hemisphere was measured from the mid-line to the inner border of the skull. Transverse cerebellar diameter (TCD) and cisterna magna diameter (CM) were measured in the suboccipitobregmatic plane of the head. The femur length (FL) was measured from the greater trochanter to the lateral condyle. For abdominal circumference (AC), a transverse section of the fetal abdomen was taken at the level of the stomach and the bifurcation of the main portal vein into its right and left branches. The anteroposterior (AD1) and transverse (AD2) diameters were measured and AC was calculated [3.14 × (AD1+AD2)/2]. The following ratios were calculated: HC/AC, HC/FL, Va/H and Vp/H.

For each of the measurements and their ratios, regression analysis was applied examining linear, quadratic and cubic models for the association with gestational age (in days). For those measurements where the standard deviation increased or decreased with gestation, logarithmic or square root transformation was applied to stabilize variance. If the quadratic or cubic terms did not improve the original linear model (an independent correlation with $p < 0.05$ and improvement of the correlation coefficient), the linear model was chosen as the best fit. Where the quadratic or cubic components did improve the model, they were included in the equation for the regression line. Equations for regression lines on transformed data were used to calculate the mean and residual SD in transformed units. To produce the reference ranges in the original units, the mean and limits of the calculated reference range in transformed units were subjected to anti-logarithmic or power transformation as appropriate.

Table 1 Biparietal diameter (mm)

Gestation	5th	median	95th
14+0 – 14+6	28	31	34
15+0 – 15+6	31	34	37
16+0 – 16+6	34	37	40
17+0 – 17+6	36	40	43
18+0 – 18+6	39	43	47
19+0 – 19+6	42	46	50
20+0 – 20+6	45	49	54
21+0 – 21+6	48	52	57
22+0 – 22+6	51	56	61
23+0 – 23+6	54	59	64
24+0 – 24+6	57	62	68
25+0 – 25+6	60	66	71
26+0 – 26+6	63	69	75
27+0 – 27+6	66	72	78
28+0 – 28+6	69	75	81
29+0 – 29+6	72	78	85
30+0 – 30+6	74	81	88
31+0 – 31+6	77	83	90
32+0 – 32+6	79	86	93
33+0 – 33+6	81	88	96
34+0 – 34+6	83	90	98
35+0 – 35+6	85	92	100
36+0 – 36+6	86	94	102
37+0 – 37+6	87	95	103
38+0 – 38+6	88	96	104
39+0 – 39+6	89	97	105

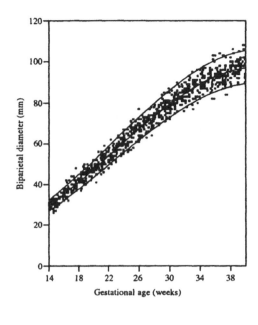

Table 2 Head circumference (mm)

Gestation	5th	median	95th
14+0 – 14+6	102	110	118
15+0 – 15+6	111	120	129
16+0 – 16+6	120	130	140
17+0 – 17+6	130	141	152
18+0 – 18+6	141	152	164
19+0 – 19+6	151	163	176
20+0 – 20+6	162	175	189
21+0 – 21+6	173	187	201
22+0 – 22+6	184	198	214
23+0 – 23+6	195	210	227
24+0 – 24+6	206	222	240
25+0 – 25+6	217	234	252
26+0 – 26+6	227	245	264
27+0 – 27+6	238	256	277
28+0 – 28+6	248	267	288
29+0 – 29+6	257	277	299
30+0 – 30+6	266	287	309
31+0 – 31+6	274	296	319
32+0 – 32+6	282	304	328
33+0 – 33+6	288	311	336
34+0 – 34+6	294	317	342
35+0 – 35+6	299	323	348
36+0 – 36+6	303	327	353
37+0 – 37+6	306	330	356
38+0 – 38+6	308	332	358
39+0 – 39+6	309	333	359

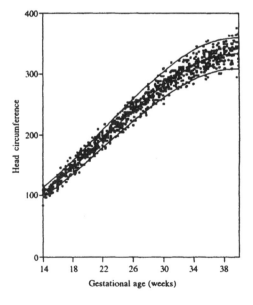

Table 3   Anterior cerebral ventricle diameter (mm)

Gestation	5th	median	95th
14+0 – 14+6	5.2	6.7	8.1
15+0 – 15+6	5.3	6.8	8.3
16+0 – 16+6	5.4	6.9	8.4
17+0 – 17+6	5.6	7.0	8.5
18+0 – 18+6	5.7	7.2	8.6
19+0 – 19+6	5.8	7.3	8.8
20+0 – 20+6	5.9	7.4	8.9
21+0 – 21+6	6.1	7.5	9.0
22+0 – 22+6	6.2	7.7	9.2
23+0 – 23+6	6.3	7.8	9.3
24+0 – 24+6	6.4	7.9	9.4
25+0 – 25+6	6.6	8.1	9.5
26+0 – 26+6	6.7	8.2	9.7
27+0 – 27+6	6.8	8.3	9.8
28+0 – 28+6	7.0	8.4	9.9
29+0 – 29+6	7.1	8.5	10.1
30+0 – 30+6	7.2	8.7	10.2
31+0 – 31+6	7.3	8.8	10.3
32+0 – 32+6	7.5	9.0	10.4
33+0 – 33+6	7.6	9.1	10.6
34+0 – 34+6	7.7	9.2	10.7
35+0 – 35+6	7.9	9.3	10.8
36+0 – 36+6	8.0	9.5	10.9
37+0 – 37+6	8.1	9.6	11.1
38+0 – 38+6	8.2	9.7	11.2
39+0 – 39+6	8.3	9.8	11.3

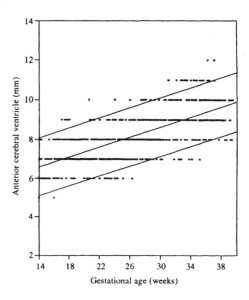

Table 4   Posterior cerebral ventricle diameter (mm)

Gestation	5th	median	95th
14+0 – 14+6	5.1	6.7	8.4
15+0 – 15+6	5.1	6.8	8.5
16+0 – 16+6	5.2	6.9	8.6
17+0 – 17+6	5.3	7.0	8.7
18+0 – 18+6	5.4	7.1	8.8
19+0 – 19+6	5.5	7.2	8.8
20+0 – 20+6	5.6	7.2	8.9
21+0 – 21+6	5.6	7.3	9.0
22+0 – 22+6	5.7	7.4	9.1
23+0 – 23+6	5.8	7.5	9.2
24+0 – 24+6	5.9	7.6	9.3
25+0 – 25+6	6.0	7.7	9.3
26+0 – 26+6	6.1	7.7	9.4
27+0 – 27+6	6.1	7.8	9.5
28+0 – 28+6	6.2	7.9	9.6
29+0 – 29+6	6.3	8.0	9.7
30+0 – 30+6	6.4	8.1	9.8
31+0 – 31+6	6.5	8.2	9.9
32+0 – 32+6	6.6	8.3	9.9
33+0 – 33+6	6.7	8.3	10.0
34+0 – 34+6	6.7	8.4	10.1
35+0 – 35+6	6.8	8.5	10.2
36+0 – 36+6	6.9	8.6	10.3
37+0 – 37+6	7.0	8.7	10.4
38+0 – 38+6	7.1	8.8	10.4
39+0 – 39+6	7.2	8.8	10.5

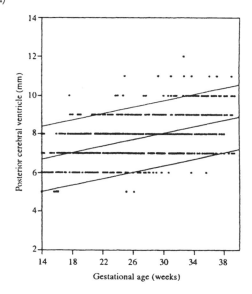

Table 5 Anterior cerebral ventricle diameter to hemisphere diameter ratio

Gestation	5th	median	95th
14+0 – 14+6	0.39	0.47	0.56
15+0 – 15+6	0.36	0.43	0.51
16+0 – 16+6	0.33	0.40	0.48
17+0 – 17+6	0.31	0.37	0.44
18+0 – 18+6	0.29	0.35	0.41
19+0 – 19+6	0.27	0.32	0.39
20+0 – 20+6	0.26	0.31	0.37
21+0 – 21+6	0.24	0.29	0.35
22+0 – 22+6	0.23	0.28	0.33
23+0 – 23+6	0.22	0.27	0.32
24+0 – 24+6	0.21	0.26	0.31
25+0 – 25+6	0.21	0.25	0.30
26+0 – 26+6	0.20	0.24	0.29
27+0 – 27+6	0.19	0.23	0.28
28+0 – 28+6	0.19	0.23	0.27
29+0 – 29+6	0.19	0.22	0.27
30+0 – 30+6	0.18	0.22	0.26
31+0 – 31+6	0.18	0.21	0.26
32+0 – 32+6	0.18	0.21	0.26
33+0 – 33+6	0.18	0.21	0.25
34+0 – 34+6	0.17	0.21	0.25
35+0 – 35+6	0.17	0.21	0.25
36+0 – 36+6	0.17	0.21	0.25
37+0 – 37+6	0.17	0.21	0.25
38+0 – 38+6	0.17	0.21	0.25
39+0 – 39+6	0.17	0.21	0.25

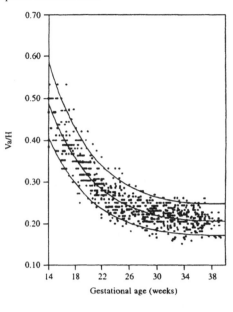

Table 6 Posterior cerebral ventricle diameter to hemisphere diameter ratio

Gestation	5th	median	95th
14+0 – 14+6	0.36	0.45	0.56
15+0 – 15+6	0.34	0.42	0.52
16+0 – 16+6	0.31	0.39	0.48
17+0 – 17+6	0.29	0.36	0.45
18+0 – 18+6	0.27	0.34	0.42
19+0 – 19+6	0.26	0.32	0.40
20+0 – 20+6	0.24	0.30	0.37
21+0 – 21+6	0.23	0.29	0.35
22+0 – 22+6	0.22	0.27	0.34
23+0 – 23+6	0.21	0.26	0.32
24+0 – 24+6	0.20	0.25	0.31
25+0 – 25+6	0.19	0.24	0.29
26+0 – 26+6	0.18	0.23	0.28
27+0 – 27+6	0.18	0.22	0.27
28+0 – 28+6	0.17	0.21	0.26
29+0 – 29+6	0.17	0.21	0.26
30+0 – 30+6	0.16	0.20	0.25
31+0 – 31+6	0.16	0.20	0.24
32+0 – 32+6	0.16	0.19	0.24
33+0 – 33+6	0.15	0.19	0.24
34+0 – 34+6	0.15	0.19	0.24
35+0 – 35+6	0.15	0.19	0.24
36+0 – 36+6	0.15	0.19	0.24
37+0 – 37+6	0.15	0.19	0.24
38+0 – 38+6	0.15	0.19	0.24
39+0 – 39+6	0.15	0.19	0.24

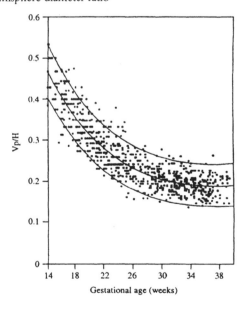

Table 7 Transverse cerebellar diameter (mm)

Gestation	5th	median	95th
14+0 – 14+6	12	14	15
15+0 – 15+6	13	15	17
16+0 – 16+6	14	16	18
17+0 – 17+6	15	17	19
18+0 – 18+6	16	18	21
19+0 – 19+6	17	20	22
20+0 – 20+6	19	21	24
21+0 – 21+6	20	22	25
22+0 – 22+6	21	24	27
23+0 – 23+6	22	25	28
24+0 – 24+6	24	26	30
25+0 – 25+6	25	28	31
26+0 – 26+6	26	29	33
27+0 – 27+6	27	31	34
28+0 – 28+6	29	32	36
29+0 – 29+6	30	33	37
30+0 – 30+6	31	35	39
31+0 – 31+6	32	36	40
32+0 – 32+6	34	37	42
33+0 – 33+6	35	39	43
34+0 – 34+6	36	40	44
35+0 – 35+6	37	41	46
36+0 – 36+6	38	42	47
37+0 – 37+6	39	43	48
38+0 – 38+6	40	44	49
39+0 – 39+6	41	45	51

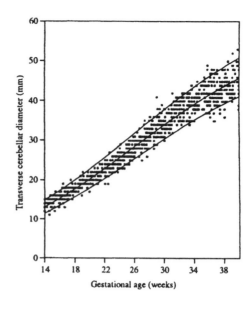

Table 8 Cisterna magna diameter (mm)

Gestation	5th	median	95th
14+0 – 14+6	1.9	3.5	5.3
15+0 – 15+6	2.1	3.8	5.7
16+0 – 16+6	2.4	4.1	6.0
17+0 – 17+6	2.6	4.3	6.3
18+0 – 18+6	2.8	4.6	6.6
19+0 – 19+6	3.1	4.9	6.9
20+0 – 20+6	3.3	5.1	7.2
21+0 – 21+6	3.5	5.4	7.5
22+0 – 22+6	3.7	5.6	7.7
23+0 – 23+6	3.9	5.8	8.0
24+0 – 24+6	4.1	6.0	8.2
25+0 – 25+6	4.3	6.2	8.5
26+0 – 26+6	4.4	6.4	8.7
27+0 – 27+6	4.6	6.6	8.9
28+0 – 28+6	4.7	6.8	9.1
29+0 – 29+6	4.9	6.9	9.3
30+0 – 30+6	5.0	7.0	9.4
31+0 – 31+6	5.1	7.2	9.6
32+0 – 32+6	5.2	7.3	9.7
33+0 – 33+6	5.3	7.4	9.8
34+0 – 34+6	5.3	7.5	9.9
35+0 – 35+6	5.4	7.5	10.0
36+0 – 36+6	5.4	7.6	10.0
37+0 – 37+6	5.4	7.6	10.1
38+0 – 38+6	5.5	7.6	10.1
39+0 – 39+6	5.5	7.6	10.1

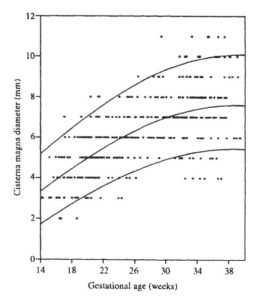

Table 9 Abdominal circumference (mm)

Gestation	5th	median	95th
14+0 – 14+6	80	90	102
15+0 – 15+6	88	99	112
16+0 – 16+6	96	108	122
17+0 – 17+6	105	118	133
18+0 – 18+6	114	128	144
19+0 – 19+6	123	139	156
20+0 – 20+6	133	149	168
21+0 – 21+6	143	161	181
22+0 – 22+6	153	172	193
23+0 – 23+6	163	183	206
24+0 – 24+6	174	195	219
25+0 – 25+6	184	207	233
26+0 – 26+6	195	219	246
27+0 – 27+6	205	231	259
28+0 – 28+6	216	243	272
29+0 – 29+6	226	254	285
30+0 – 30+6	237	266	298
31+0 – 31+6	246	277	310
32+0 – 32+6	256	287	322
33+0 – 33+6	265	297	334
34+0 – 34+6	274	307	345
35+0 – 35+6	282	316	355
36+0 – 36+6	289	324	364
37+0 – 37+6	295	332	372
38+0 – 38+6	302	339	380
39+0 – 39+6	307	345	387

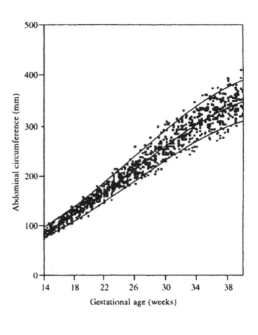

Table 10 Head circumference to abdominal circumference ratio

Gestation	5th	median	95th
14+0 – 14+6	1.12	1.23	1.33
15+0 – 15+6	1.11	1.22	1.32
16+0 – 16+6	1.10	1.21	1.31
17+0 – 17+6	1.09	1.20	1.30
18+0 – 18+6	1.09	1.19	1.29
19+0 – 19+6	1.08	1.18	1.29
20+0 – 20+6	1.07	1.17	1.28
21+0 – 21+6	1.06	1.16	1.27
22+0 – 22+6	1.05	1.15	1.26
23+0 – 23+6	1.04	1.14	1.25
24+0 – 24+6	1.03	1.13	1.24
25+0 – 25+6	1.02	1.12	1.23
26+0 – 26+6	1.01	1.11	1.22
27+0 – 27+6	1.00	1.10	1.21
28+0 – 28+6	0.99	1.09	1.20
29+0 – 29+6	0.98	1.08	1.19
30+0 – 30+6	0.97	1.08	1.18
31+0 – 31+6	0.96	1.07	1.17
32+0 – 32+6	0.95	1.06	1.16
33+0 – 33+6	0.94	1.05	1.15
34+0 – 34+6	0.93	1.04	1.14
35+0 – 35+6	0.92	1.03	1.13
36+0 – 36+6	0.91	1.02	1.12
37+0 – 37+6	0.90	1.01	1.11
38+0 – 38+6	0.89	1.00	1.10
39+0 – 39+6	0.88	0.99	1.09

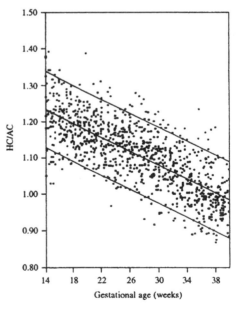

Table 11 Femur length (mm)

Gestation	5th	median	95th
14+0 – 14+6	14	17	19
15+0 – 15+6	17	19	22
16+0 – 16+6	19	22	25
17+0 – 17+6	21	24	28
18+0 – 18+6	24	27	30
19+0 – 19+6	26	30	33
20+0 – 20+6	29	32	36
21+0 – 21+6	32	35	39
22+0 – 22+6	34	38	42
23+0 – 23+6	37	41	45
24+0 – 24+6	39	43	47
25+0 – 25+6	42	46	50
26+0 – 26+6	44	48	53
27+0 – 27+6	47	51	55
28+0 – 28+6	49	53	58
29+0 – 29+6	51	56	60
30+0 – 30+6	53	58	63
31+0 – 31+6	55	60	65
32+0 – 32+6	57	62	67
33+0 – 33+6	59	64	69
34+0 – 34+6	61	66	71
35+0 – 35+6	63	68	73
36+0 – 36+6	64	69	74
37+0 – 37+6	66	71	76
38+0 – 38+6	67	72	77
39+0 – 39+6	68	73	78

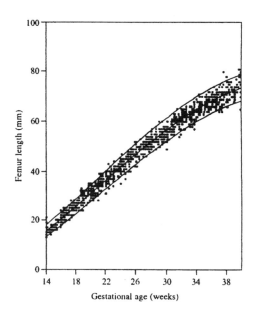

Table 12 Head circumference to femur length ratio

Gestation	5th	median	95th
14+0 – 14+6	6.08	6.55	7.05
15+0 – 15+6	5.81	6.28	6.76
16+0 – 16+6	5.59	6.04	6.52
17+0 – 17+6	5.40	5.84	6.31
18+0 – 18+6	5.23	5.67	6.13
19+0 – 19+6	5.09	5.53	5.98
20+0 – 20+6	4.98	5.41	5.85
21+0 – 21+6	4.88	5.31	5.75
22+0 – 22+6	4.80	5.22	5.66
23+0 – 23+6	4.74	5.16	5.59
24+0 – 24+6	4.69	5.11	5.54
25+0 – 25+6	4.65	5.06	5.50
26+0 – 26+6	4.62	5.03	5.46
27+0 – 27+6	4.60	5.01	5.44
28+0 – 28+6	4.58	4.99	5.41
29+0 – 29+6	4.56	4.97	5.40
30+0 – 30+6	4.54	4.95	5.38
31+0 – 31+6	4.52	4.93	5.36
32+0 – 32+6	4.50	4.91	5.34
33+0 – 33+6	4.48	4.89	5.31
34+0 – 34+6	4.45	4.85	5.27
35+0 – 35+6	4.41	4.81	5.23
36+0 – 36+6	4.35	4.76	5.17
37+0 – 37+6	4.29	4.69	5.11
38+0 – 38+6	4.21	4.61	5.02
39+0 – 39+6	4.12	4.51	4.92

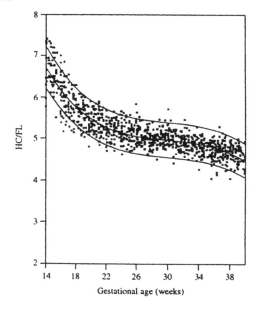

WEB SITES PROVIDING USEFUL INFORMATION FOR PRENATAL DIAGNOSIS

- The fetus on line: http://www.thefetus.net/
- Medline: http://www.ncbi.nim.nih.gov/PubMed/
- Online Mendelian Inheritance in Man:
  http://www3.ncbi.nlm.nih.gov/Omim/searchomim.html
- Prenatal Diagnosis of Congenital anomalies: http://www.prenataldiagnosis.com/

Index

T - #0617 - 071024 - C0 - 246/189/8 - PB - 9780367399689 - Gloss Lamination